*"Medicine can restore the health of
a human but cannot generate it.
Health is born from within the being."*
Radha Gopalan, MD

ENDORSEMENTS FOR *SURVIVAL*

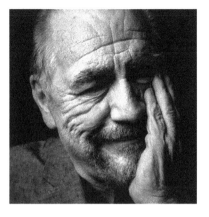

Brian Denis Cox
Emmy and Golden Globe award-winning actor

Radha Gopalan's follow up book to his brilliant *Second Opinion, Survival* is a wholly unique testament and manual dedicated to the consciousness of health and greatly elevates the confusion between disease culture and health culture. A riveting do-it-yourself plan embracing the true paths to health. A first class must-read epistle!

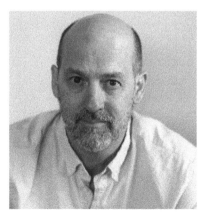

Anthony Edwards
Golden Globe award-winning actor

Dr. Gopalan has done it again. He has found the light and hope from having lived the realities of the darkness. Drawing from a wide range of experiences as a Heart Transplant surgeon, an ayurvedic, acupuncture and Yoga teacher, he shares the many ways we can empower ourselves to be responsible for our health. There is lightness and joy that comes through his openness in teaching. He shows us how important it is to connect deeply with our universal spirit, and to practice from unconditional love, as opposed to the fear-based tradition of "healthcare" being "disease care". We can follow the power of spirit with the support of well thought out "self-care". We can practice the principles he shares every day by believing that we can make a change. *Survival* is a book of hope.

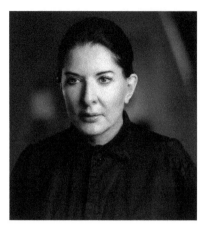

Marina Abramović
New York Dance and Performance award-winning performance artist
Portrait of Marina Abramović, 2018
Ph: Carlo Bach

Radha Gopalan's *Survival* has been released in what is possibly the best moment in human history. Reading this book is different than any other publication, which, when you are done, you put it on the shelf and forget about it. This is a guide that will come in handy at any moment of your life.

– MUST READ!

– MUST PRACTICE!

– MUST SHARE WITH OTHERS!

This is not just a book. This is invaluable knowledge in book form.

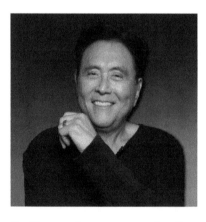

Robert Kiyosaki
International Best-selling author, entrepreneur, financial educator, and founder of Rich Dad Education

Dr. Radha Gopalan has been my cardiologist, personal physician, teacher, and friend since 2006. His lessons are always about the differences between health and medicine. In his new book, Survival, Radha teaches us to make finer distinctions and better understand the path to good health. Ever since the COVID-19 pandemic of 2020, I have become even more proactive regarding my health—changing my diet, losing weight, and exercising vigorously. I do this because Radha has taught me well: a vaccine may protect me from COVID…but a vaccine is not health.

BATTLING PANDEMICS, EPIDEMICS AND DISEASE

SURVIVAL

A PHYSICIAN'S GUIDE TO HEALTH AND BEING YOUR OWN HEALER

RADHA GOPALAN, MD

HEART TRANSPLANT CARDIOLOGIST, ACUPUNCTURIST & YOGA INSTRUCTOR

SURVIVAL:
A Physician's Guide to Health and Being Your Own Healer
by Radha Gopalan, MD
1. OCC000000 2. MED004000 3. MED034000
ISBN: 978-1-949642-77-3
EBOOK: 978-1-949642-78-0

Cover design by LEWIS AGRELL

Printed in the United States of America

Authority Publishing
11230 Gold Express Dr. #310-413
Gold River, CA 95670
800-877-1097
www.AuthorityPublishing.com

TABLE OF CONTENTS

PART III
How do I do it?
8 TRANSFORMATIONAL RULES

INTRODUCTION

Survival depends on success. Success means a win.

A Question

Do you want to be on the winning side or the losing side?

Everyone wants to be a winner—but winning in the realm of health is a challenge for most of us. No one really knows how to even define health. This was evidenced by the global catastrophe of the 2020 pandemic, when the fear of falling ill made us all ask: "Would I survive the virus?" It was more of a pandemic of fear than a pandemic of disease. Everyone knows what *disease* is, but there is worldwide confusion about what constitutes *health*. As a result, being healthy is elusive for most of us.

Nevertheless, many people erroneously view themselves as healthy, though most people I've asked couldn't even define health. It's therefore not surprising that we're becoming an unhealthy population that relies on outside factors and entities to maintain our health. When the outside entity fails, we fail. Not a smart way to ensure survival.

Is there a way to ensure our survival before a health crisis, such as a pandemic, or a heart attack, stroke, liver disease, kidney disease, lung disease, cancer, etc. tests us? The answer is yes.

A Global Medical Failure

The year 2020 will be known as the year when the entire world experienced a surge of death, panic, pain, and poverty. For the first time in the history of the US, a status of disaster was declared for the fifty states and five territories—all caused by an invisible enemy. Even regular diseases that we encounter daily are invisible enemies, not just a virus of a pandemic. Every nation in the world attempted to fight this agent of destruction while it hijacked our bodies leading to the death of millions and the collapse of the world economy. It was named SARS-CoV-2 (Severe Acute Respiratory Syndrome-Coronavirus 2), and it caused the pandemic of COVID-19 (Coronavirus Infectious Disease – 2019).

The attack was a surprise. No one knew exactly where the virus came from or how it jumped from primarily animal hosts to humans or how it got the capacity to not just infect, but to kill. The bug was a killing machine that nobody knew how to fight. This novel virus that had never attacked humans before dumbfounded scientists. As the virus devastated our lives, its qualities remained an enigma; all we knew was that it was three times as powerful (virulent) as a known flu virus. There are several theories of its inception, such as: engineered virus, modified virus, natural transmission from animals to humans, biological warfare, and even nonscientific considerations such as God's fury and the end of the world. No matter how we look at it, the global death was real. *The message: Human health is fallible.*

Medical professionals around the world struggled to understand the nature of the illness and the phenomenon it created. No treatment existed, no vaccine was available, and nobody knew how to prevent its spread. It was a failure of the global medical field, leading to death and devastation unprecedented in this generation. No matter the country—whether developed or emerging—healthcare professionals, scientists, and governments were stumped. The best weapon they devised to overcome the enemy was a preventative measure called "social distancing" which placed the entire responsibility on us. Risk aversion was the best strategy we could come up with. *The message: Modern medicine is fallible.*

The name "modern medicine" in this book is used to describe the medicine promoted and practiced by health care systems across the world. Whereas the name "traditional medicine" is used collectively to denote medical practices of what is known as complementary and alternative medicine or medical practices of different religions, cultures, tribes, and ethnicities.

Neither modern nor traditional medicine had an immediate answer to the problem. "Stay home and stay healthy" was a formula designed to promote social distancing and to slow the virus' spread. In other words: preventing physical contact with each other for fear that one of us may harbor the virus and transmit it to others. Many people perceived government lockdowns as a violation of human rights. The entire world embraced itself with fear. The best we accomplished with this tactic was slowing the spread of the virus—that's it! But it did nothing to help you win if you became infected. *The message: The healthcare system can fail us.*

What is clear, and what was openly expressed during the pandemic, was that the above formula was created by medical professionals and widely adopted by governments across the globe to buy time. Time was needed, they said, in order to identify and manufacture weapons against the invisible enemy. These weapons included vaccines, diagnostic tests, antivirals, antimalarial, ventilators, etc. Experts agreed on one common theme: We must understand the disease so that we can treat it. This is the theme, understanding the disease and not the person suffering from the disease, that drives modern medicine. Sadly, hundreds of thousands died during this period of medical inadequacy. *The message: Relying on the medical systems of the world is not smart.*

A Lesson

The collective system failed you and me!

Those infected were isolated and looked upon as if they were lepers. Definitive help was not available; therefore, we couldn't rely on anyone or anything. Our only hope was a hospital professional who didn't know what to do other than to isolate, give supportive measures, and watch, as the patient either progressed toward survival or death. It was up to the patient to declare success or failure. In other words, the healthcare professionals and the system depended on our health status for success or failure. *The message: Doctors and health systems rely on you for success or failure—you are the medicine. It is true for all diseases at all times but just got amplified during the pandemic.*

People who weren't infected were left to tend to themselves during the lockdown period. Non-infected persons had to make do with the basic essentials and avoid contact with the virus. *The message: At the end of the day, the effort is our responsibility.*

Medical practitioners, irrespective of modern or alternative training, could not come up with life-saving treatment fast enough, other than supportive care. State and local governments couldn't help. Family members couldn't help. Schools and universities closed. Transportation was reduced, leaving people isolated and stranded. Doctors refused to meet with patients one-on-one. Disease-altering elective medical testing and procedures were prohibited, or in some states illegal, as they were considered "non-urgent." This strategy allowed other chronic diseases to progress and advance unabated. *The message: Even a responsible person, faithfully tending to their illness, can be let down by the collective system during a catastrophe.*

Places and activities that boost our emotional wellbeing were prohibited. Playgrounds closed. Restaurants closed. Places of worship closed. Health clubs closed. Poverty increased. Unemployment rates climbed to previously unknown levels. Stock markets crashed. Fear of violence among populations increased, and as a result, gun sales skyrocketed. The system as we knew it collapsed!

Each of us was left living in fear, without the tools to combat the enemy if contact was made. The only solution was to hide from possible exposure—a fair tactic, but the enemy proved infectious enough to find some of us. The system that we rely on takes our health for granted and it failed us when we needed it most.

The lesson: It is not smart to rely on the system or any other outside entity to help us in times of crisis. The smarter choice is to *rely on ourselves, and use the system and outside entities as tools rather than crutches for success.*

It's amazing how many of us don't employ this simple strategy. We wishfully think that the problem will go away, that "It won't happen to me," and we go back to our old ways, until another catastrophe gives us a wake-up call—the cycle repeats. There is a saying: A wise person learns from other people's mistakes, only fools wait to learn from their own.

A Realization

The other side of the coin is that not everyone that caught the virus died! Four distinct groups of people emerged out of those that came into contact with this enemy. The first are those that developed severe illness and were unable to overcome the virus, rapidly dying—they lost the fight. The second are those that contracted the virus, developed mild to moderate illness, were hospitalized, and successfully recovered—they fought and won with support. The third group consists of those people who contracted the virus, developed mild symptoms, and recovered without hospitalization—they fought and won without support. The fourth group are those that came into contact with the virus and didn't even know it—they won without a fight. We called them "asymptomatic," and they had an inherent ability to defeat the virus. *The message: The ability to overcome diseases is unique to each human.*

At the time of writing this on April 25, 2020, the ratio for those who recovered versus those that died is 4:1 according to a Worldometer report. This illustrates that for every five infected persons, one of them didn't have an inherent ability to win the battle even with supportive treatment. The recovered group had some inherent ability to win, and the asymptomatic group had an even stronger inherent ability. The statistic is staggering. You may be curious about what this inherent ability is. *The question: What is it that the survivors possessed that the deceased did not?*

In science and medicine, the result of this inherent ability is called "differential response." Differential response means that people respond to insults, such as a disease, in different ways that is unique to each individual. In other words, no two individuals respond the same way to an identical insult. What underlies this differential response is our unique inherent ability to overcome an insult. This inherent ability, the subsequent differential response, and how to harness this ability is the focus of this book.

All of us have an inherent ability to win over illness. It has everything to do with the natural tendency of survival. The pandemic shed light on the strength and vulnerability of this inherent ability. It made us realize that this inherent ability is unique to each of us, and doesn't depend on any outside factors or entities, such as the medical system or government. It also showed us that most of us aren't working to cultivate this inherent ability. For those who survived, it was a wake-up call. *The realization: Everyone continues to forget the most lethal weapons we possess—the human mind & body!*

The pandemic came as a massive wave that swept across the world and forced us to re-examine our belief system and understanding of health and disease. In this book, we'll find narratives of how to understand "health" as understood by both modern and traditional medicines. We'll come to understand why modern medicine cannot simply make us healthy, and why relying on modern medicine alone is unwise. More importantly, we'll learn how to change our lives so that we're prepared to be on the winning side, whether we're fighting acute illnesses like the pandemic, or chronic diseases that afflict and kill us slowly. Both, acute and chronic diseases, are invisible enemies to humanity.

Loss of life, no matter how you look at it, is devastating. I've sat by the side of dying patients countless times and witnessed the devastation it causes not just to them, but to their families and caregivers as well. There are three types of people when it comes to death. There are those that know death is imminent and make peace with it. There are those who understand that death is imminent and fight it. And then there are those that don't even realize they're dying—we don't want to belong to this group. This is one area where ignorance is not bliss, unless we don't mind dying prematurely. I've had the opportunity to stand at the bedside, look into their eyes, and have a conversation with all three kinds of people. There's a story behind those eyes that is beyond the scope of this book to tell. However, the core message is contained in the book. Suffice to say that natural death is expected, but premature death is not. It can, and should, be prevented.

Modern medicine does not have the tools, money, and time to engage in this debate. I chose to try to understand this discrepancy. You are currently holding the fruit of those reflections in your hand. Reflections on this, along with my experiences with patients, revealed an astounding phenomenon that we all ignore: modern medicine totally misses the concept of health while excelling in delivering disease care. The majority of modern medicine's effort is consumed by the business of disease care—what bothers me more, is the refusal of humanity to acknowledge it. How many people have to die before we recognize the truth that is hiding in plain sight?

How about you? Do you want to take the chance with an inadequate medicine to save you, or do you want to understand how the survivors survived? It's a wake-up call for all of us. This book is about individual empowerment in health, and how to function outside of the system.

· ·

Formula to remember:
Winners rely on themselves; losers rely on the world.

· ·

PART I

WHAT IS HEALTH, ANYWAY?

6 MYTH-BUSTING VIEWS

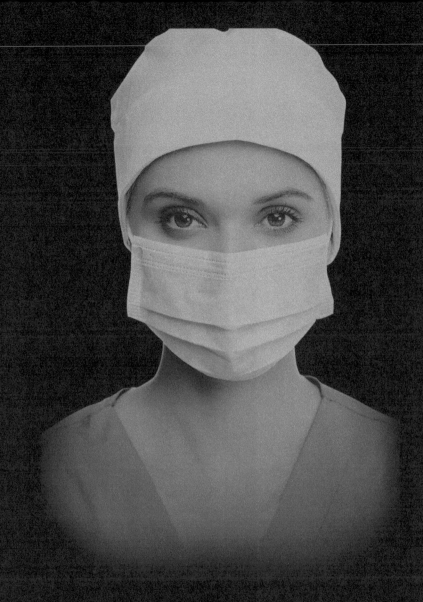

INDIVIDUAL'S VIEW

WORLD'S VIEW

MEDICINE'S VIEW

BODY'S VIEW

SPIRIT'S VIEW

WINNING VIEW

CHAPTER 1

Individual's View: A Myth

The Illusionist

For most people, the concept of health is an illusion!

Simply put, most of us think we know what health is, but we really don't. When asked what health is, we struggle to come up with a clear answer. Health is conceived as just the absence of disease because it's easy, simple, and disease is tangible. True health is like a diamond in the rough: hard to recognize with its presence and positive qualities masked by daily distractions. Looking through the prism of disease prevents the true understanding of health. It is wrong!

For example, if you are thirty years old and think you're healthy because you haven't been diagnosed with any diseases, you're wrong. If you're sixty years old, take medications for one or two medical conditions, and think you have your health back in absolute, you are wrong too. Why is it wrong?

A better question is: How do the thirty- and sixty-year-olds know they are healthy? The answer is … they don't. There are no exact tools to measure health because there's no unit to measure it by. It cannot be quantified. Individual health is qualitative—it's subjective, which makes it easy to misinterpret. Perception is treated as reality—we believe what we want to believe. The human body is a very complex system of mechanisms consisting of trillions of cells. These mechanisms work together in synchrony toward one purpose: survival. They're active every second, minute, hour, day, week, month, and year. The total duration of their continued living constitutes our life span. These cells and their mechanisms don't go to sleep when we do—if they went to sleep, we'd die.

The thirty-year-old is waiting for symptoms of disease to appear so that it can be quantified. The sixty-year-old appreciates the quantitative difference in the existence of symptoms before and after treatment, and thinks that this improvement means health is restored. Both are an attempt at quantification of health through symptoms of disease. Both are stuck in an illusion that they're healthy. That is, until a new symptom suddenly appears, a diagnosis is made, and a medication is prescribed. All of a sudden, you've lost your health. Just like that!

If we were infected with COVID-19, we could have died or survived. If we suffer from a chronic disease, we may live with ill-health. Once we've been diagnosed with a disease, we have to confide in our family, and maybe in our friends. We have to inform our health insurance, and pay increased premiums. We have regular doctor's appointments and take medications. Life as we know it has changed, just as the COVID-19 pandemic rapidly changed countless lives. Should we allow ourselves to suffer under an illusion that alters the path of our lives? Isn't that ignorance?

When I say we must rely on ourselves, I mean that we should do so with a proper understanding of health, not with deceptive thinking. *The first step is being true to our self. Deceiving our self is the biggest mistake we can make.* This is true not only when it comes to health, but also for life in general.

The Illusionist at Play

Meet one of my patients, Mr. Illusionist: a handsome, forty-eight-year-old who was sent for consideration of heart transplant for end-stage heart disease. He looked younger than his age. He was a successful accountant employed by a major US banking system. Medically, all the tests and investigations revealed that his heart was dying and had no strength to support his body. Pills were not enough to bolster his circulation because his heart was still too weak. He needed two different medications administered through his veins (intravenous route) to be kept alive. Most of his other organs were functioning at a slower rate, but blood tests indicated that their function was within normal range. This meant that the other organs were salvageable if the heart problem was fixed. All attempts to wean him off the two intravenous medications failed.

Mr. Illusionist had been feeling ill for six to twelve months, but hoped his symptoms would improve without intervention. He didn't seek medical attention, as he didn't believe he was unhealthy.

Thinking that the ill feelings would magically improve after months of silent suffering were an illusion and a denial of one's own experience. Thus it was a self-deception.

During his hospital stay, Mr. Illusionist was able to eat, sleep, and sit in a chair in the intensive care unit. He was only able to walk as far as the bathroom, located in the corner of his room, and then back to his bed. He spoke rationally, but was unrealistic in thinking that he was "fine." If you'd seen him sitting in the chair and talking to you, you wouldn't think he was dying.

Mr. Illusionist was presented with the option of heart transplant, as well as mechanical circulatory support (a mechanical heart pump) to keep him alive until a suitable heart became available. He refused these recommendations. Instead, he requested to be discharged home, so that he could heal in a comfortable environment. His mind could not accept that his body was dying.

Patients are normally not discharged home while on two intravenous medications—it's not practical or safe. Mr. Illusionist was presented with the option to be discharged to hospice care on both medications. He accepted, and was transferred to hospice. The next morning, Mr. Illusionist passed away. The body died, taking with it a functional, active, young, and educated mind. But the illusion of the mind was the true culprit in allowing the body to die.

Self-deceivers are Losers

If we fall for the deception around us, and deceive our own self, there is no winning. Health is misconstrued and misrepresented worldwide. Healthcare systems misrepresent it. Media misrepresents it. Insurance companies misrepresent it. Governments misrepresent it. None of this is intentional; they simply don't understand what health is, and misrepresentation follows.

Nevertheless, it is deceptive. Doctors aren't trained to make us healthy; they're trained to treat diseases. We then misunderstand and misrepresent the idea of health to ourselves. We live in ignorance until the day that disease comes knocking on our doors. When that happens, we may still play the illusionist by being in denial. We give a multitude of explanations as to why this happened. Again, we look outside ourselves to understand the phenomenon that caused the disease. If we cannot find an answer, we play the victim and pick up the "Why me?" tune. We don't look within ourselves and ask the tough questions: "What did I do—or not do—that contributed to this?" Or "Where did I miss the warning sign?" Few people do.

What we, as individuals, know about health is what our society represents to us. School doesn't teach about health; there's no curriculum for true health at school. When I was in school, the health curriculum consisted of children spending time in the playground. Current health courses in the US consist mostly of information on illegal drugs, nutrition, and sex education, but not in the context of true health. Many parents don't teach their kids about health because they were not taught. Religion doesn't teach about health. Doctors don't teach about health. We learn from what is around us, but what is around us is misguided. This form of observation is the worst way to learn about health. Because there is no quantifiable way to understand health, and because it is subjective, it's easy to misrepresent. Listen to the commercials telling you what to do to be healthy. If you really pay attention, you'll realize those commercials are not about health, they're about surrogates of health, or about disease.

What's around us deceives us, and we in turn deceive ourselves by living in a health bubble with a false sense of security. When the COVID-19 pandemic hit, even those that were in this health bubble ran scared. They didn't have confidence in their own health. Why? They weren't confident because the sense of security wasn't real; it was an illusion. That feeling of safety is a distraction from a deeper fear within us. That fear is about confronting the truth and about denial of the truth. We deny that our health is slowly declining over the years. We live with this false sense of security until disease presents itself and health is lost.

In fact, even young, healthy doctors ran scared during the pandemic. I saw some of my colleagues change their behavior overnight—it was laughable. I worked at the hospital every day during the pandemic and witnessed how absurd the environment at work became. When fear struck at the core of their being, their pretention melted away. With that melting, the emptiness of our sense of security was revealed. People became scared, but a lot of the people wouldn't admit it, even to themselves, let alone to others.

The COVID-19 pandemic demands we reexamine our understanding of health. Light was shed on health as it's understood today, and its misguided nature was revealed. For most people, this type of realization happens when a serious crisis occurs, like a heart attack or stroke. The pandemic was a wake-up call delivered rapidly and simultaneously to millions around the world, catching us off guard. For many of the "apparently healthy people" that died, health, as they understood it, didn't help. My experience as a physician is the same. Most of my patients, just like Mr. Illusionist, died when their perception of health was clouded by the illusion of wishful thinking. The wrong perception became their individual reality. *Dying is not a good way to learn that we had the wrong idea about being healthy.* If we want to be on the winning side, it's time to break free of the illusion and take charge of our own health.

CHAPTER 2

World's View: Misdirected

The Concept of Real Health is Hidden in the Hype

E very hundred years or so, a pandemic like COVID-19 causes a wave of devastation throughout the world and sheds light on several aspects of human life. As we've already explored, by affecting millions of people, the pandemic illuminated the falsity of our current understanding of health. This level of disillusionment has a tendency to force our attention toward the disease side of the coin, and we forget to look at the other side of the coin. Because our current understanding of health is firmly tied to the presence or absence of disease, we wait for a disease like COVID-19 to open our eyes. That is, if you are a survivor.

The "wait-and-see" attitude is the byproduct of our erroneous ideas about health. The smart thinkers tend to be proactive and prepared. The wise approach is to direct our attention to the other side of this pandemic coin, the side that's usually not "hyped up" by the media, government, and medical professionals. This is the side of the survivors, and you want to ask, "What protected them?" Winners develop the habit of making objective assessments of situations prior to taking action. Others are guided by reflexive action and blind trust based on what the environment feeds them.

In the week of June 27, 2020, the top health advisor to the White House came on national television and said, "I have never seen a virus causing a disease where forty percent of infected people have no symptoms, some have mild symptoms, some have severe symptoms, some get hospitalized, some have to go on ventilators and recover, and others go on ventilators and can't survive." This was the "top guy" in our medical system addressing the people, and it's an example of the unbalanced focus on the death caused by the pandemic while ignoring how the survivors survived. The entire world talked about the characteristics of people who died or could die but no mention of the characteristics of people who are survivors.

The 2020 pandemic differentiated five groups of people among the world's population (1–5 below). If we consider only those people that came into contact with the virus, there are four groups of people (2–5 below). Each of these groups has a story to tell about health. If we look closely, these stories reveal the uncut diamond—the *health reserve* of an individual to ward off disease. The ability of the human body to mount a response to fight illnesses, when required, is called the *health reserve* of an individual. Health reserve is not just concerned with the immune system fighting infections or inflammatory conditions but also includes the reserve to overcome other chronic illnesses like diabetes, high blood pressure, heart disease, liver disease, kidney disease, etc.

Group 1: Those that did not come into contact with the virus—the untested. These people didn't have to fight, as there was no contact. The consequence of this is that they don't know the level of their health. When the number of hospitalizations was declining across the country, and people were emerging from isolation, there were reports of new cases among those who'd successfully self-isolated during the peak. The question is: how did these people get infected despite self-isolation? Successful isolation does not guarantee immunity to the disease; it minimizes the chance of coming into contact with the agent of disease. Once the rules were relaxed, the unhealthy people, even though successful in isolating themselves during the peak, contracted the disease. Those that were unhealthy in this untested group became ill with the virus and fell into Group 3, 4, or 5 below. Coming into contact is a chance event, which is a statistical phenomenon. Taking action, just like social distancing, can influence statistical probability. Who survives and who dies after making contact is determined by the degree of health reserve an individual possesses—not chance.

Group 2: Those that came into contact with the virus but did not develop any symptoms—the unaffected. These people had the strongest health and immune system; the virus couldn't even start a fight. These individuals had significantly high health reserve. The enemy was powerless against these people; it was as if the virus didn't exist as far as they were concerned. The virus could inhabit their bodies, but not invade. The health status of this group is preventative, and guards them from threats from the outside world (like the SARS COV-2) or from within the human body (like chronic diseases). This is the best health status to be in. However, it's important to note that, despite their individual health, members of this group carried the virus and possibly infected others.

Group 3: Those that contracted the virus and developed mild symptoms that resolved without hospitalization—the affected strong. These individuals' health reserve was just enough to thwart the fight early, before any significant damage was done. The health status of this group was not optimal, but it was strong enough to mount a fight that ended with little damage to the person. If we consider health as a spectrum, this group falls in the middle between healthy and unhealthy. As a result, they were able to rebound and rebalance with no significant permanent damage, even though they developed mild symptoms.

In my line of work as a physician, I don't come into contact with the people in the groups described above. Modern doctors don't know exactly what to do with them. The absence of disease disables the modern physician's ability to care for a person's health. Once disabled, modern medicine and its providers fall back to advocating "health maintenance." Unfortunately, as we've discussed, this idea of health is misconstrued, and it's impossible to maintain something that we don't have a solid understanding of. As far as modern medicine is concerned, if there are no symptoms or diagnosable disease, you are "healthy."

Group 4: Those that contracted the virus, developed symptoms requiring hospitalization, but left the hospital alive—the affected weak. These individuals didn't have enough health reserve to finish the fight with the virus alone; they needed extra support. With supportive care provided by the medical system, they overcame the disease. Without that extra support, they may not be alive today. Their health reserve alone was not sufficient to win the fight. You can think of it as like bringing an allied country's troops to fight our war. The modern medical system was an ally to this group of people in fighting the disease. Remember, modern medicine only provided supportive care; there was no proven medication to treat COVID-19. The inherent health reserve of their body was sufficient—with a little extra support—to win the fight, even without a targeted medication to kill the virus.

Group 5: Those that contracted the virus, developed symptoms requiring hospitalization, lost the fight, and left the hospital in a body bag—the affected dead. The individuals in this group had depleted their health reserve to a point that even with full support provided by modern medicine, their bodies could not fight off the disease. This level of depleted health reserve is expected in the elderly or those with multiple medical conditions. However, it's strange that even those without any other disease (labeled healthy) ended up succumbing to the pandemic. What's more, even children have died. Therefore, age alone does not universally guarantee good health or health reserve to fight off illnesses. There are a lot of young people who believe that their youth will protect them from dying of any disease. Even worse, the young feel that it won't happen to them—that is, until it does. For some, it's terminal.

A Reversed Outcome

The following story is a true and personal illustration of Mr. and Mrs. Ronas who I cared for during the pandemic. They were both in their early sixties, who observed self-quarantine recommendations in their home. The husband was an active, "healthy" gentleman with no prior diagnosis and no prescription medications. He walked three to four miles a day, three times a week, in addition to working full time. His partner was a housewife who suffered from hypothyroidism (under-functioning thyroid gland) and was taking replacement medications. She led a sedentary lifestyle, except for during household activities.

A little more than two weeks after the husband self-quarantined from work, he developed fatigue, tiredness, altered taste, and lack of appetite—but no fever. He consumed a liquid diet in hopes the symptoms would go away on their own. Believing he was healthy, he didn't seek medical attention. Each year, he underwent the required medical examination provided by his employer. The annual exam suggested that he was healthy—no disease was ever identified. But, three days after his symptoms began, his heart stopped. Paramedics arrived at his home, resuscitated him, and he was taken to the hospital. In the hospital, he received the maximum amount of supportive care that can be provided by modern medicine in a developed country. Five days after admission, he died. On the day of his death, his COVID-19 results came back positive.

His wife, however, had symptoms of fatigue and tiredness that lasted three days. She also cared for her illness by consuming a liquid diet in the hope of self-resolution. By the time the husband went into cardiac arrest, the wife had recovered. After the death of her husband, the wife tested positive for SARS COV-2 but had no symptoms at the time of testing. Irrespective of the absence of symptoms, she was treated with oral medications without requiring hospitalization.

Both husband and wife lived in the same home. The husband was declared a healthy man by modern medicine, while the wife would be considered unhealthy due to her under-functioning thyroid and replacement medications. They were both of the same race and culture, and weren't poor. During the pandemic, modern medicine across the world declared that people with underlying medical conditions are at higher risk of developing complications due to COVID-19 than those without. By this token, the outcome for this couple should have been reversed. Instead, the wife belonged to Group 3 and the husband to Group 5. Modern medicine failed to properly assess the health reserve of these two individuals, because it used the wrong concept of health, and consequently, the wrong tools. They were labeled incorrectly.

These misdirected medical assessments make us pause and think as to how much reliance can be placed on modern medicine when it comes to our health reserve. Measuring health by the presence or absence of disease is a crude strategy. What was it that allowed the "unhealthy" wife to escape unscathed, but the "healthy" husband to perish? It was the difference in their *health reserve* that is not captured by modern medicine's assessments.

While modern medicine doesn't successfully measure health, it does inform us if we have a disease or not. Medical professionals are very familiar with the concept of health reserve, but that concept operates in their subconscious, because they predominantly handle disease, not health. We, as physicians, frequently struggle with this in practice. I've seen patients die that we believed would do well. I've also seen patients that we declared to be high-risk (less likely to live through treatment) proceed like champions without any complications.

The presence or absence of a medical diagnosis doesn't equate to the body's ability to fight other illnesses. Though the presence of a pre-existing illness may impair the overall ability to overcome another disease (like COVID-19), it's by no means an indication of the health reserve that any given individual has against an insult. No two individuals of the same gender and age, and suffering with the same disease, necessarily have the same health reserve.

The Diamond in the Rough

Health is not about one or two variables like age, diet, exercise, or presence or absence of disease. It's about multiple life variables coming together, which gives us a certain degree of ability to overcome disease. *This ability is directly proportional to health reserve.* The more health reserve one has, the better the ability to fight disease.

The *status of health* is an estimate of the health reserve one has. The status of our health determines if we're going to be winners or losers when tested by an insult—like the coronavirus. The difficulty with health status is that it's intangible—there's no tool to measure it. This is the very reason modern medicine relies on tangible and measurable variables (such as the presence or absence of disease) to declare one as healthy or unhealthy, and it's why I've described the people in the different groups above as strong, weak, or unhealthy. But there are tools to identify our *health status* and to recognize a decline in health reserve.

The amount of health reserve a person has varies, as illustrated by the different groups during the pandemic. The health reserve varies in subtle ways, not just among a group of people, but also among individuals within the same group. This calls not only for individualized assessments of health, but also for individualized efforts to maintain health. As a result, achieving and maintaining health is up to each one of us—the individuals, not the world's medical systems or any other entity. That effort is our own.

CHAPTER 3

Medicine's View: Disease-oriented

A Misdirected Focus

As a heart transplant specialist who cares for patients suffering from end-stage heart disease, my job is to implement the most advanced medical and surgical therapies. The purpose of treatment is two-fold: to give patients the opportunity to live longer, and to improve their quality of life. This is based on the premise that the presence of disease tends to shorten our life span.

All of my patients have heart disease in one form or another. Most of them not only have heart disease, but also other diseases such as diabetes, high blood pressure, high cholesterol, kidney disease, etc., and thus have multiple medical diagnoses. These patients are offered the best medical and surgical therapies that modern medicine can supply. They're sometimes prescribed multiple medications for each diagnosis. While polypharmacy presents a problem of its own, the real problem is that instead of focusing on the person with the disease, modern medicine focuses on the disease.

I have seen patients who would've died if left untreated, recover and walk out of the hospital thanks to the marvels of modern medicine. Paying attention to disease is not a bad thing, but pretending to take care of health is.

I do this every day in my practice. This is how I was trained. When it comes to treating diseases, modern medicine excels and is second-to-none. The significant and rapid advancements made in the past few decades have benefited humanity across the world. The achievements made by scientists working tirelessly to advance our understanding of disease are unparalleled. I'm proud to be associated with some of the scientists in this era. Nevertheless, the main focus is on treating the disease, as illustrated below in Figure 3.1.

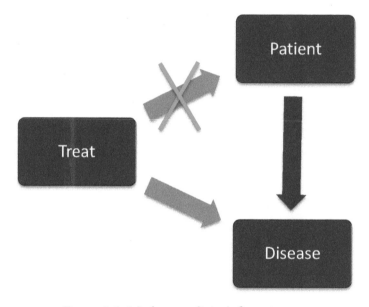

Figure 3.1: Modern medicine's focus is away
from the person and their health.

Because we've defined good health as the absence of disease, we've allowed disease to creep into our definition of health. As marvelous as modern medicine is at combating acute and chronic diseases, it's insufficient in combating the recurrence of disease and the burden of it. As seen during the pandemic of COVID-19, modern medicine is helpless in this regard, leaving us to fend for ourselves. Those with the best health reserve survived and those with the worst health reserve perished.

A Disabling Concern

Mr. Artist, a patient of mine in his eighties, had recurrent headaches, and presented to the emergency room with these headaches twice. Both times a CAT (computed automated tomography—an expensive test) scan of the head was negative for any abnormalities to explain the headaches. The first time, he was admitted for observation, which means he was watched overnight in the hospital to observe any changes in his condition. He was then sent home with pain pills.

The second time, he was sent home with a pill for pain and a pill for spasms of the neck muscles to treat the headache. He returned to the clinic for follow-up with the same debilitating headaches. He had arthritis of the neck with muscle spasms due to many years of being hunched over while he worked. The combination of aging with long periods of uncorrected poor posture caused an imbalance in the way his musculoskeletal system worked. As a result, he developed arthritis of the upper back, shoulders, and neck.

From a modern medical perspective, the appropriate intervention would be to give one medicine for the arthritis, and another for the muscle spasm, with additional instructions for physical therapy. No aspect of this strategy gives the patient any control over the situation. I asked my elderly patient to continue taking mild pain relievers, and I additionally taught him very simple yoga exercises for his shoulders and neck during one of our forty-five-minute visits. He went home and practiced these exercises daily for just fifteen to twenty minutes. To learn the yoga exercises, he neither had to come back three times a week, nor return at all for three months. He now had control.

The pain medications helped him to initially execute the exercises comfortably. If the pain weren't controlled, he would have been discouraged from continuing the yoga exercises—no one wants to go through more pain to get rid of existing pain. More importantly, he was empowered to engage his spirit in the process.

Since that day, he's had no headaches, is off of his pain medications, and continues to enjoy life. At this point, he is mentally, emotionally, and socially balanced, and free of pain. He's not optimally healthy, but has at least reached a new balance with regard to his primary problem of arthritis. From here he can slowly move toward even better health. His other option was to continue the Band-Aid approach of taking pain medications forever.

Medications mostly mask the underlying problems. Medications are designed to counter an internal process of disease that has already started. For example, when we take antibiotics to treat an infection, the medication is intended to weaken or kill the bacteria. With the bacteria weakened, the body is able to overcome and defeat the bug. The antibiotic does not strengthen the underlying weak health condition that initially allowed the bacteria to invade us. Antibiotics temporarily tip the balance of the battle in favor of our body so that the body is allowed time to strengthen to eliminate the bacteria. Strengthening the underlying health is our responsibility. The same rule applies to chronic diseases. Remember, during the COVID-19 pandemic, the world did not have any medications to treat neither the virus nor the process triggered by it. Hundreds of thousands died. Most medications are not designed to eliminate the reason the disease was triggered but to curb the progress of a particular disease process. That's why there's no single medicine to treat all different diseases.

Medications are studied, researched, and developed to control the progression of disease in the hope of alleviating or minimizing symptoms and prolonging life. Disease is diagnosed by identifying symptoms and signs in a person. These only occur further down the road of a disease process, long after the disease started inside our bodies and mind. As a result, by the time we diagnose a disease, the process has already been advancing for some time. That's why it's unwise to wait until symptoms develop to proclaim our health status. Likewise, relying totally on medications to treat an already-present disease is also a bad idea. Our personal engagement in the process and utilization of all available tools is essential. The book *Second Opinion: Eight Deadly Diseases* by this author describes several modalities that serve as our tools for this very purpose.

A Clear Sight

Mr. Artist is a very simple example of a successful combination of modern medicine with the power of a human being. The health reserve of a person is totally under the control of that person; it is not under the control of modern medicine. We should learn to use, but not rely on, modern medicine. Relying on it can result in catastrophic outcomes, as is what happened for those that perished during the pandemic. Unknowingly, they weren't prepared; the medical system could not take care of them.

When we empower human beings to engage their own self, their health reserve increases. In fact, when we prescribe only medications, we actually further disable the patient; we add to their disability by disempowerment. The optimal formula is enabling, not disabling. The reason for success in this patient's case was actually due to simultaneously treating the disease and the patient, as illustrated in Figure 3.2. It was teaching him to do the yoga exercises, restoring his faith in himself, helping to correct the posture, and giving him total control (as opposed to just the medications) that made the difference. I was not taught this combination in medical school—it came from my experiences as an acupuncturist and a yoga teacher.

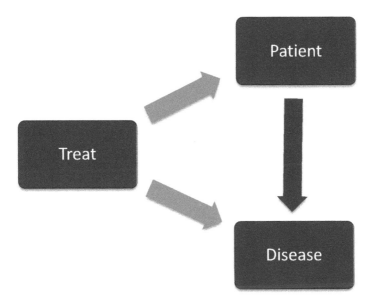

Figure 3.2: Simultaneous focus on the disease and the patient.

Understanding Disease

In medical school, I was taught how to recognize, diagnose, and treat diseases. Medical students are taught about normal physiology (function of the human body) and anatomy (structure of the human body), but not about health. Students are taught what is normal and not introduced to *what actually drives* that normal structure and function or how that "normal" should be maintained—they are only taught what normal looks like.

The reason they are taught what normal should be is to recognize when disease alters the normal. Learning about diseases is called pathology (abnormal structure and function of the human body). Students are taught all the features of disease and the altered internal body processes that lead to the development of disease. Then they're taught how to diagnose these diseases by identifying altered structure/function, symptoms, and signs that suggest a particular disease. What they aren't taught is how to recognize when the disease process begins inside a human body before symptoms develop. No one knows; therefore, we ignore it. Physicians are trained to be experts in abnormality, not normality. But health is about normality.

Disease is so prevalent that we have come to accept it as part of our life. We've all heard of diseases, know someone that's been diagnosed with one, and maybe have one ourselves. Despite this, we identify disease only when it comes knocking on our door with a symptom or sign—we don't actively go looking for it. But diseases start within our body weeks, months, and years before we develop recognizable symptoms. Disease is actually a manifestation of declining health reserve.

A Life-threatening Concern

October 11th, 2006, was an eventful day. While running on the treadmill in the early morning, I felt a slight chest discomfort. I stopped and thought for a few minutes about what it could be. Being a cardiologist, I was aware that discomfort from the heart—called "angina pectoris"—is usually brought on by exertion, and is relieved by rest. The pain should also be further increased by more exercise.

I decided to test this, and continued to exercise. The discomfort went away instead of further increasing. The first occurrence of angina is labeled as "unstable angina," indicating that it can progress to a heart attack. It can also wax and wane. Likewise, continued angina without exertion for more than twenty to thirty minutes is also called unstable angina, and indicates a possible heart attack.

The discomfort returned when I was taking a shower, and continued at a rating of about a two out of ten in intensity (in this scale, zero means no pain and ten means the worst pain one has ever experienced). Since there was no change in the intensity of pain with exertion, I decided to go to work and test myself at the office.

First, I had to rule out a heart attack. After four hours of chest pain, I did an ECG (Electrocardiogram—a test that captures the electrical activity of the heart and enables doctors to diagnose a heart attack or insufficient blood supply to the heart) and a blood test to determine if there was heart muscle death. Both tests were negative. I continued to work through the day with the pain, which remained at an intensity of two to three out of ten throughout.

At the end of the workday, fear set in. Not wanting to go home without a diagnosis, I went down to the emergency room at about 4:00 p.m. and talked to the physician about my symptoms. He and I agreed that it did not appear to be angina, but decided to rule out an alternate, more benign explanation of acid reflux.

I swallowed viscous Lidocaine (a numbing medicine in gel form) and waited at the emergency room to see the result. If my condition was reflux, then the viscous Lidocaine should relieve the pain within minutes of swallowing it. But the pain remained!

I admitted myself to the emergency room and repeated the same tests I'd done earlier in the day. This time, they turned out positive for a small heart attack. The on-call cardiologist was not convinced that it was a true heart attack, considering my young age, physical capacity, endurance, and lack of risk factors. He wanted to monitor the situation on medical therapy until the next morning to see how the condition evolved. I, however, insisted on having an immediate cardiac catheterization.

This test is an invasive procedure involving the placement of catheters through the main artery in the groin or wrist, which are then advanced to the heart. Dye is then injected into the blood vessels that give blood supply to the heart and reveals if there's a blockage. A blocked artery should support the diagnosis of a heart attack.

The catheterization revealed that one of the three blood vessels to my heart was completely blocked, cutting off blood supply to the bottom part of my heart. Two stents were placed inside the blood vessel to keep it open.

Clouded Focus

The problem isn't just misdirected ideas of health; it's clouded focus too. Young people do get heart attacks—that is the nature of being unhealthy. It was devastating when it happened to me. I had been testing my heart by running three miles a day, without any symptoms, up until then. I'd followed every bit of the advice I gave my patients regarding diet, exercise, and compliance with regular medical check-ups, because I had a family history for heart disease. I had followed everything that modern medicine recommended. I practiced Eastern philosophies such as yoga and meditation, and took additional nutritional supplements. I've also had acupuncture treatments and taken homeopathic tinctures on and off throughout my life. My body mass index (BMI) for the prior fifteen years had remained at twenty-three to twenty-four (in modern medicine, this is a healthy body based upon height and weight).

Yet, Mr. Cardiologist had a heart attack!

With the exception of having a family history of early-onset heart disease, I was doing everything that modern medicine recommended to prevent a heart attack. I didn't smoke, I didn't use recreational drugs, and I consumed alcohol only occasionally during social events. Yet there it was: a cardiologist with a heart attack.

My cardiologist was puzzled, and so was I. Needless to say, I was treated just like anyone else would be in a modern hospital. After the stents were placed, I spent three days in the hospital, and was then discharged home with four appropriate medications, and was told that I was "good to go."

I was labeled with a disease and sent home with medications, just like Mr. Artist with his headaches. I was told to eat low-fat, low-salt foods, and engage in regular exercise after a few weeks (even though I was already doing all of this, even before the heart attack). These are the recommendations I would have given to any of my patients when they suffer a heart attack.

However, these recommendations were useless to me, as I was already following them for many years. After my personal experience, I somehow felt as if modern medicine's attention to the entire event was incomplete. None of the modern medical concepts explained why this event occurred.

I just did not understand why this happened to me after diligently following what I preached. After all, I am a cardiologist myself. If I would not rely on modern medicine for health, would you? My knowledge of Eastern medicine didn't help me understand how this event occurred either.

It's well known in the medical field that a human has to have disease of the blood vessels to the heart itself to suffer the most common form of a heart attack. The vessels supplying blood to the heart are called the coronary arteries, and the disease of these vessels is called atherosclerotic coronary artery disease.

Coronary artery disease does not materialize in one day; it's a slow process. In fact, research shows that blood vessels of ten-year-old children already have initial features of atherosclerotic disease. Unbeknownst to me, I had the disease progressing during my teen years and my twenties without symptoms. That's why I warn teens and young adults that youth does not guarantee the absence of disease (more on this in Chapter 13).

On the other hand, not every teen and youth has an undiagnosed disease. Some may, and others may not. Explaining this lack of uniformity is beyond the scope of this book, but identifying who may have a disease and who may not is also very difficult. Modern medicine fails in this aspect too. This reinforces why each one of us has to be diligent about health, and be our own champions.

I relied on modern medicine's indicators to assess the status of my health just like Mr. Ronas did. My thinking was clouded by the knowledge I possessed. I was looking for disease because that's what everything around us is informing us to do. That's why I was looking for symptoms, and waited until symptoms developed, to assess the level of my health. Believe it or not, this is the same knowledge I share with my patients, and I cannot help but wonder how it clouds their thinking process. The misdirection is so strong that even medical people get sucked into it. Imagine how misdirected people outside the medical world can become.

My cardiologist told me, "This is what happens when you have a family history, even though you did not have any other well-known risk factors." He was trying to explain the unexplainable. He couldn't just say, "I can't explain what happened to you." As physicians, we're expected to explain events that occur in medicine. If we cannot, we are at risk of being perceived as incompetent.

I have known several people that had a family history of heart attacks, but did not have a heart attack themselves, and I've known several people who did not have a family history, yet had a heart attack anyways. Similar statements can be made about other chronic diseases as well. We could ignore this discrepancy and move on, as most of us (physicians and patients) do. But this is a very powerful discrepancy; it speaks for the individuality of health.

It's similar to the medical system failing to explain how young people died during the COVID-19 pandemic. We all agree, if you are old or have other diseases, you are at high risk of death with COVID-19, but we cannot explain it the same way for the young who died. No two people are the same.

CHAPTER 4

Body's View: Dichotomous

The Power of the Human Body

The most powerful personal health tool in the world is our own body. The human body is a resilient and pliable structure. It can withstand a great deal of abuse, while still functioning to maintain balance in the face of these abuses. It is the most physically tangible and appreciable possession of a human being, and a priceless gift that we possess.

We all started off as a single, powerful cell with only one purpose—survival. That single cell evolves into multiple cells, which work in synchrony to form our body. As we grow and get caught up in the hype of the world, we lose sense of how powerful and resilient our bodies are, and we abuse them. When the body tells us that it's malfunctioning via subtle symptoms and signs, we ignore it. We continue the abuse and expect the body and its cells to self-repair, which they do, but not for long.

As time progresses and the abuse continues, the ability of these cells to repair and return toward normal function declines. This ability depends on how much health reserve the cells have left in them. When the body finally falls apart in an area, such as the heart, lungs, or kidneys, we're labeled with a disease.

The wake-up process happens at the time of a disease being diagnosed like how we felt during the COVID-19 pandemic. Some of us personally became infected, while others watched as friends and family fell ill. By that time, it was too late to prevent disease, but not too late to establish a new balance for the cells that fell apart. Why? Because the human body is resilient, if proper attention is given to it. But who repairs, and who dies, depends on the health reserve of each particular person, as we discussed in Chapter 2.

It's estimated that an average human body's cell count ranges between thirty to thirty-seven trillion. Starting off as a single cell and ending up with thirty to thirty-seven trillion is a very complex task. Cells increase by a process called "cell division." They don't just divide; they also differentiate, meaning different cells become specialized to perform different functions.

To help us understand this, consider a football team as one unit, just like our body. Within that team, there are players that specialize in performing specific functions, such as the quarterback, linebacker, wide receiver, running back, etc. These players did not originally start off specialized; they became specialized. In our body, we call these players heart, brain, liver, skin, kidneys, and so on. These are called organs, and there are approximately seventy-eight of them in the body.

If the members of the football team don't play in a seamless fashion, the team loses the game. If our organs don't perform seamlessly with vigor against adversaries like the coronavirus, our body loses the fight—game over.

Sometimes, a football player is injured and all other players have to rise to the challenge and play harder without the injured player. Playing the game under this circumstance is more difficult, and requires more energy from each remaining individual. If the other players have enough reserve, they stand a chance to win. If not, they lose.

In our body, when one or two organs don't function optimally due to a pre-existing disease, the rest of the body has to put up more energy to fight additional adversaries, like the coronavirus. That's why the world's governments and medical scientists warned us that if we already have a disease, we're at a higher risk of dying from COVID-19. If our health reserve is already being utilized to fight an ongoing chronic disease, we don't have maximum reserve for fighting an additional attack.

A football coach has to train the team in not only the skills and strategy of the game, but also in developing the reserve to be used in times of need. If we want to be winners, we need to train our body to have health reserve ready to access at any time, like having money in a savings account.

Those of us who simply go through the motions of the day and hope everything will be all right stand to lose. This mindset is like training your team just enough to be able to play the game. That is not a winning team. We are the coaches of our own health, not modern medicine. A winning body needs active training and coaching. Are we ready to be the coach our body needs? If we are, we win. If not, we lose. Loss in this case means suffering, underperformance, disability, accelerated aging, and even death.

Imagine how trillions of cells can function seamlessly with each other, take our abuse, and still survive. Perhaps, the smartness of a cell outperforms the smartness of our mind. Some organisms on our planet, like bacteria, are comprised of only one cell. They are adaptive, but not as smart as the cells of an evolved organism like humans. That is, unless we make our body's cells less smart than the adaptive ability of a bacterium, parasite, or virus. That's exactly what happens when we don't care for our bodies and continue to lose our health reserve. The problem is; while we're making ourselves less smart, the single-celled organisms are constantly evolving into better-adapted beings.

How is it that we cannot fight single-celled organisms after beginning as one, smart cell, and then developing into multiple, smart cells in our body? It's due to the environment that we create for our own cells in the body. An abused body has a poor environment and poorly-functioning cells, while a well-maintained body has the best environment and excellently-functioning cells. A poorly-functioning body is disease-prone by virtue of the low level of health reserve. An excellently-functioning body is disease-resistant by virtue of having ample health reserve to overcome disease.

The Seed or the Soil – A Great Debate of Dichotomy

"The Seed or the Soil" was a debate concerning the most important factor for the development of disease in humans. In nineteenth-century France, two giants of scientific medicine, Louis Pasteur (1822–1895) and Claude Bernard (1813–1878), proposed radically different paradigms for the development of disease in humans.

Louis Pasteur, a chemist and the father of modern medicine's germ theory, proposed that germs (seeds) are the sole reason that humans develop disease. His work provided the cornerstone of modern medicine's advances in the treatment for infectious diseases. Based on Pasteur's theory, scientists and pharmaceutical companies have developed medications against bacteria (antibacterial), viruses (antivirals), and parasites (antiparasitic) that modern medicine uses profusely today.

The opposing theory proposed by Claude Bernard was not popularized, and was nearly lost to history. Claude Bernard, a physiologist and colleague of Pasteur, argued that the "terrain" (soil) is more important than the seed. He proposed that germs could only succeed in infecting people who are already sick in some way.

Bernard and his colleague Béchamp together argued that not everyone exposed to the same germ would develop a disease. During this time, the infectious disease known as cholera was very prevalent in Europe. Apparently, Claude Bernard drank a glass of water containing cholera-causing bacteria, without developing the disease, and thus proved his theory to his pupils (Rediger, 2020).

Bernard's theory never advanced beyond this experiment with regard to infections because it's easier to identify and develop medications against the germ (a tangible source of disease), than to discover the intangible power of the terrain to resist infection. Because it's more difficult, there's no financial gain in the latter. Furthermore, the power of the terrain lies within us, and is immeasurable. It cannot be harnessed by an outside entity or by taking an elixir. The terrain is the personal responsibility of each individual. This terrain theory later became the foundation of modern physiology.

What Claude Bernard meant by "terrain" is the internal environment of the human body. He proposed that a well-balanced environment is strong enough to ward off infections. Conversely, an unbalanced environment is predisposed to contracting disease when exposed to a disease-causing agent. This theory of constant internal balance underlies the entire study of physiology in modern medicine, and is called "homeostasis" in physiology.

The Oxford English Dictionary defines homeostasis as "the tendency toward relatively stable equilibrium between interdependent elements, especially as maintained by physiological processes" (www. oed.com). The problem is, there's no formula, either in modern medicine or in traditional medicine, for assessing and quantifying this internal balance that can be monitored over time. Therefore, health became immeasurable. It's up to us, as individuals, to understand and assess our own health, and this is described in Part II and III of this book.

The Merit

Louis Pasteur's germ theory has merit. Germs do, in fact, cause infectious diseases and kill people. Sometimes they kill people in isolation, sometimes in an epidemic, and sometimes in a massive pandemic like COVID-19.

The terrain theory of Claude Bernard has merit, too. We learned in Chapter 2 that not everyone exposed to the coronavirus developed the disease or died. We were able to identify four distinct groups of infected people, and saw that it was the terrain that made the difference between those groups, despite them being exposed to the same virus. Here is what we know that provides merit to the role of "terrain" in infectious diseases:

1. Not every human that's exposed to an infectious agent develops disease or dies from it, as seen in pandemics and epidemics throughout history.

2. Germs can be either symbiotic or pathogenic to humans, depending on the environment. There are trillions of germs, bacteria, and parasites that live in our intestines and on the skin without causing any disease. Biologists from the Weizmann Institute of Science reviewed all available literature and came up with an estimation of these organisms: a "reference human being" (twenty- to thirty-year-old male, seventy kg weight, 170 cm height) harbors about thirty-nine trillion bacterial cells. That's more cells than what our own body is made of. Yet, the organisms and our body live together harmoniously. Some of these organisms protect us from attack by other, more virulent germs—this is the "symbiotic relationship." However, these normally harmless germs can sometimes cause disease when our body's resistance is reduced. Our resistance is reduced when our optimal internal homeostatic balance is disrupted. This, for example, occurs frequently in hospitalized patients. When patients are sick from one or more diseases, and their bodies' internal balance is disturbed, they become infected by the very organisms that live harmoniously within us.

3. The body's response to infection is individualized, depending on the health reserve of the individual. The terrain (internal environment) and its balance are unique to each individual. Although our bodies are made up of the same cells and structures, our internal environments have unique signatures, just like our genetics and fingerprints. That's why there were different responses to the same virus among those that got sick (Groups 2, 3, 4, & 5 in Chapter 2) during the pandemic of 2020.

Legend has it that on his deathbed, Louis Pasteur is said to have admitted that, "the germ is nothing, the terrain is everything (Cowan and Morall, 2020). However, in my experience, both the germ and the terrain are equally important.

Because both the germ and the terrain are the opposing components that underpin the dynamics of what we are discussing—balance. Both the seed and the soil count when it comes to health and disease.

Based on the two giants' debate, it appears as though terrain is aligned with health (but not disease), while germ is aligned with disease (but not health). Our "health" system, by virtue of focusing on disease, has advanced our solution to germs by successfully discovering medications, antidotes, and vaccinations. However, the same "health" system has miserably failed to advance actual health, because the system is blind to it.

Acknowledging the power of the germs as responsible for causing disease and ignoring the power of our health reserve to resist such causation is misleading. These concepts were confused right from the beginning, when Louis Pasteur and Claude Bernard started this debate. Germs have their own internal environment, just like we have our own internal environment. The purpose and unending focus of the internal environment in germs and humans alike is constant rebalance from disbalance (a process called homeostasis), caused by adverse agents, and more importantly, *survival.*

Germs get the advantage when an individual's health reserve to resist is low, because the individual is vulnerable enough for the germ to invade and propagate.

We call that person unhealthy.

On the other hand, germs are powerless to an individual whose terrain is strong.

We call that person healthy.

Germs invade us not because they want to; it's a survival instinct that is simply carried out when the germ finds a weak host—a suitable environment to thrive. Likewise, our cells' survival instinct will attack the germs and keep them suppressed. It's a fight between two organisms, and their internal environments contain their weapon of war—health reserve. The strength of the health reserve depends on how well-balanced the internal environment is, and the organism with the most balanced internal environment wins. As Charles

Darwin stated: it's survival of the fittest. *Being the fittest is not about being strong, it's about being adaptive.*

Therefore, both the germs and the terrain are important aspects regarding health, and survival depends on the respective strengths of each. *Health and survival are not the same, but are directly proportional.*

For our body, being healthy is a matter of maintaining balance with the goal of survival. The body focuses on constantly re-establishing and maintaining balance of the internal environment for the purpose of averting or overcoming any threat to that goal.

Health, therefore, can be conceived of as an organism's *ability* to withstand and overcome an adverse force on its internal environment, and its *ability* to re-establish and maintain the balance of that environment.

The Deficiency

The reason for the departure from "healthcare" to "disease care" partly resides in the absence of a specific definition of health. Current, commonly used definitions of health are flawed. The Oxford English Dictionary defines health as, "the condition of being sound in body, mind, or spirit especially: freedom from physical disease or pain." Apart from the comment about physical disease, the rest of the definition is very esoteric. Most people have trouble with the tangibility of this definition. Based on what we understand about health so far, the above definition is empty. It tells us what a healthy person looks like, not what health is. What we've come to understand about health from previous chapters would never be possible to grasp by reading the above definition, even if you read it multiple times!

In 1948, the World Health Organization (WHO) made a courageous and ambitious decision to define health as, "a state of complete physical, mental, and social well-being and not merely the absence of disease or infirmity" (Sartorius, 2006). This definition, while drawing the main focus away from the presence of disease or infirmity, still does not provide any tangible idea of what health is. It also removed the spiritual (and in my opinion, very important) component of a human being. It's still flawed in regard to defining health.

European medical professionals recognized the flaw in the WHO's definition of health and called for a new definition. A 2011 British Medical Journal (BMJ) article by Huber et al. proposed health as, "the ability to adapt and self-manage in the face of social, physical, and emotional challenges" (Huber, 2011). They recognized that there are several people who have chronic diseases, and yet have found a way to maintain robust physical, mental, and emotional wellbeing—as illustrated earlier by Mrs. Ronas who survived the coronavirus, despite having underlying medical conditions (Chapter 2). In fact, the definitions of health made by both the WHO and the Oxford English Dictionary have resulted in the medicalization of health, while giving no insight as to what health looks like or how to measure it. The European definition comes very close to what we've learned from previous chapters, but it still excludes an important, and perhaps the most powerful, component of human beings—the spirit.

CHAPTER 5

Spirit's View: Energetic

The Power of Healing

The world of medicine cannot exist without the spontaneous power of the body to heal. Medicine, whether modern or alternative, exists only to fill the gap in the body's natural ability to heal. For example, when we cut ourselves, the cut heals with little help from us. I sometimes tease my surgical colleagues that they wouldn't have a job if the body couldn't heal itself. The incisions we make on patients wouldn't close, infection would set in, and the person would die—this is a powerful truth that we don't realize often enough. The entire medical world is built on this foundation of self-healing, and serves the body by helping to re-establish its balance.

When a cut is incurred on the surface of the skin, the integrity (homeostasis) of that part of the skin is disrupted. The disrupted skin rebalances itself via healing mechanisms to serve the ultimate purpose of the body—survival. If the skin doesn't heal itself, the wound serves as an entry point for infection-causing organisms that can affect not only the local area, but also the entire body (if the body's health reserve is weak). If infection sets in, this can lead to disruption of the homeostasis of the entire body, thus placing the person at risk of dying. Therefore, the natural tendency of the body is to heal in order to survive.

The Law of Nature

When I was a kid, I wanted to be a pilot. I was drawn to the uniform, the stature, and the awe of flying a plane. Conquering air seemed like a marvelous achievement that was worthy of pursuing, but I became a physician instead. As an adult, I still wanted to learn how to fly a plane, so I started taking lessons. My first lesson was in a small plane. After climbing to a certain altitude, the instructor stalled the plane, because the first thing you need to learn as a pilot is how to recover from a stall. My heart rate and blood pressure skyrocketed and I started sweating.

The instructor asked, "What's wrong?"

I said, "We are going to fall."

I thought I was going to die.

The instructor calmly reassured me that, "The airplane wants to fly, that's how it is designed."

In other words, the natural tendency of the plane is to fly; it will only fall if we disrupt the airplane from its natural course. The wisdom behind those words stayed with me forever.

On another occasion, I was a passenger on a flight from Philadelphia to Phoenix. The "fasten seat belt" sign came on, and the pilot announced that we were headed for turbulence. I buckled my seat belt and braced myself. As we entered the turbulence, my heart rate and blood pressure started climbing. I closed my computer, emptied my glass of water so that it wouldn't spill, and death-gripped the armrest. The passenger beside me turned to me and smiled.

He said, "You seem tense."

"I don't like turbulence," I replied, "because it feels like it is a prelude to the plane falling and crashing."

He smiled again and said, "The plane wants to stay up in the air. The movement of the plane you feel is expected; it's aerodynamics. You only need to worry if the plane stops moving in response to the turbulence."

Later, I learned that I was sitting next to a pilot. Since then, I am thankful that the plane moves the way it does during turbulence. When we harness nature, we should be prepared to obey the laws of nature. Much like the tendency of a plane to fly, the law of nature for the human body is to stay healthy, because health is directly proportional to survival.

Just as the plane is designed to respond to turbulence, the body is designed to respond to insult (i.e. heal). Healing is a natural response of a living organism in order to survive. Similarly, just like the plane is designed to stay in flight, the body is designed to maintain homeostasis of its internal environment. The cells, organs, and tissues work synchronously to maintain balance for continued survival. That is the purpose of any organism, and it's no different for a human.

All purposes have a drive behind them. A drive is a force that continues to feed an action in order to accomplish its purpose. In humans, that force continuously feeds our instinct to survive, and encourages the body to maintain balance 24/7. We are born with that power. That power—that force—feeds our instinct for healing and survival, and is the "Spirit." Therefore, the spirit powers the spontaneous healing of human beings. Spirit determines our longevity.

The Spirit

Every single-celled organism in the universe has the instinct to survive. The same applies to viruses and parasites, too, as well as for multicellular organisms like humans. There is a spirit giving rise to intelligence behind that instinct in all of them. The cells have a code to decipher this intelligence, and they follow that code to survive. This code is embedded in their DNA. Sophisticated cells have sophisticated codes, and simple cells have simple codes.

Within a single cell are its organelles, and a medium in which these organelles function. When a cell dies, the organelles can no longer maintain proper function, and they're broken down. If a cell is preserved upon its death, we can examine the structure of these organelles and study them. However, they cannot function after death. What is needed for function and what infused life into the cells has left the cells, even though the physical structure of organelles and DNA were preserved. What departs at time of death is generally accepted as spirit. Attempts to identify and quantify the spirit have not been successful. It's not the organelles or the DNA that make cells function. It is the spirit. It is like a computer. The hardware and software of the computer itself cannot operate or function without electricity. When the power is turned off, the computer can be preserved but not the function. Like the software of the computer, DNA is only the software that programs a cell's function, and organelles are the hardware that carries out those functions. But neither the DNA nor the organelles can function without a force to animate them; the cell needs a force to be alive. That force is called *vital-force. That vital-force originates in our spirit.*

In modern medicine the strength of this vital-force is measured as vital signs. The vital signs that indicate the balance of our vital-force are the blood pressure, heart rate, respiratory rate, and temperature. In acupuncture the vital-force is called the "Qi" (pronounced "Chi"). All traditional medicines originating from different ethnicity and culture recognize this force and have their own name to describe it.

Spirit on the other hand, is an abstract concept, but it's an absolute requirement for life, as it provides power for the instinct to survive. Being alive, from the body's perspective, requires maintenance of the internal environment. In other words, the body needs to maintain enough health reserve to ward off adverse forces of external and internal origin and keep the internal environment at optimal balance.

We have seen that without the spirit, cells cannot balance the internal environment, even if they have the DNA coding for that function. Therefore, spirit is an integral part of the optimal maintenance of balance within us. This balance determines our health reserve. The more balanced an organism, the healthier that organism is. The less balanced an organism, the less healthy it becomes.

If the spirit does not adequately fuel the cells, maintaining balance becomes inefficient. In other words, if cells' vital-force is reduced, they cannot function well; they cannot maintain an optimally-balanced state. Their health reserve is reduced, and the cells become unhealthy. When cells become unhealthy, the organs become unhealthy and the collective body becomes unhealthy. Finally, when spirit is completely depleted, death occurs. It's easy to see why spirit is an integral part of health—a truth unrecognized in the world's perspective of health.

What Death Teaches Us

I have delivered babies and have sat next to a countless number of dying patients. I have been with, and talked to, many patients in their last few days and hours of life. There are two occasions in life where the spirit makes its biggest impact. The first moment is at birth—its entry point. The second is at death—its exit point. In between, the spirit appears irrelevant to most of us because of the world's distractions.

The fact is, we take the spirit for granted, until it is slowly depleted and unable to fuel our health. At that point, we become vulnerable to disease, either acute or chronic, and desperately try to regain the internal balance. By that time, the strength of spirit we are left with is not enough to rebalance us. The disease, if acute, kills us fast (like COVID-19), and if the disease is chronic, it kills us slowly (like diabetes or high blood pressure). If one has no disease, we die slowly of old age, due to the spirit slowly being spent.

No matter how we look at it, the spirit gives life, and is a separate entity from the body and its internal environment. Irrespective of being separate, the spirit permeates all the cells, and gives them power to function. The spirit is not the same as the body. The body, after death, can be preserved, but it cannot function without the spirit, which leaves at the time of death.

We all know that countries of the world estimate health status by measures to assess the burden of disease, mortality, and subsequently the average life span of their population (Thacker, 2006). Even we, as humans, wrongly think that disease is associated with shortened life. Health is not associated with our life span; health is associated with the spirit. Life span depends on the level and strength of spirit we possess. Weak or diminished spirit equates to short life, even if we have an otherwise healthy body with a well-balanced internal environment. Strong or elevated spirit equates to long life, even if we have a diseased body. The problem is we have no way of measuring spirit. We can only feel it, and have a sense of how strong or weak it is. Even feeling the spirit is difficult for most of us because we do not know how to recognize it. We have to be trained to do that.

Previously, in Chapter 2, we identified different groups of people with different levels of health reserve. Likewise, there are three scenarios that illustrate the existence and intricate involvement of the spirit, as a separate entity, with our health and longevity.

Three Ways to Die

Scenario 1: Sudden removal of spirit

Consider a young person who is healthy and leading a normal life. If that person commits suicide, the organs of the body are abruptly damaged to a point of no return. The spirit is no longer able to animate the organs due to loss of coordinated function, and the body loses its spirit. The body and its cells will preserve their inherent ability to function for a brief period. If medical help arrives in that brief period, our modern medicine can resuscitate the cells, which revives their function and keeps the organs functioning artificially. This young person can be kept artificially functioning for a period, until the cells slowly lose their inherent vitality and stop functioning permanently—a process we call organ dysfunction and decay.

If we remove the organs of this person quickly enough and place those organs in a new, living medium (a body where the spirit still exists), the organs will then continue to function, fueled by that new person's spirit. This is what happens in organ transplant. That is how I am able to stay in the business of heart transplant.

Organ transplants are performed all across the world. Most organs are transplantable, such as: heart, kidneys, lungs, liver, pancreas, cornea of the eye, intestines, skin, etc.

After a person dies, we assess the level of function of these organs and determine if they are good enough to be transplanted. In other words, if they have enough of their residual health reserve left to continue living once placed in a new medium where a continuous flow of spirit is assured.

Next, the organs that are deemed well-functioning are donated. All of the organs don't get transplanted into one person; they are donated to different recipients, dying due to dysfunction of a particular organ. These recipients, therefore, have at least some level of spirit and good function of other organs. This allows the transplanted organ to survive and support the bodily function in concert with the other organs. This illustrates that spirit and body function are separate entities, but work cooperatively for health and longevity; they are intricately intertwined for this purpose.

The moral here is: a healthy body with optimal health reserve is suddenly ripped of the spirit. This suggests two phenomena. First, optimal internal environment and health reserve does not guarantee longevity—we also need the spirit for longevity. The spirit can be extinguished at any time, and when it is, life concludes. Second, if the organs are in optimal condition, they can continue to function for a long time if introduced to spirit again.

I have had heart transplant patients living as long as thirty-two years with a transplanted heart. Therefore, spirit and body are separate entities, but they depend on each other to keep an organism alive.

Scenario 2: Excessive expenditure of spirit

Consider a forty-year-old person with obesity, diabetes, high blood pressure, and heart disease. These invisible enemies constantly drain the internal environment of the person. I call these diseases "invisible enemies" because that is the nature of their pathology. They don't announce themselves right from the beginning. We only diagnose them when they produce symptoms, and by that time, it's already too late. These diseases start well before (months, and sometimes, years) symptoms develop, and long before we're able to diagnose them.

We either know someone who's diagnosed with one or more of these diseases, or we suffer from them personally. These chronic diseases are constantly disrupting the balance of the internal environment—the terrain. The internal environment is continuously addressing this persistent disruption and trying to rebalance. This tireless attention to fighting the disease not only diminishes our health reserve, but also depletes part of the spirit that powers the health reserve. As a result, we don't have the maximum amount of health reserve and spirit available to us to fight battles with infections like COVID-19. That is why the WHO and the United States Center for Disease Control (CDC) announced that people with existing diseases are at higher risk of dying from COVID-19.

Even in the absence of infection, the body is excessively spending its spirit to battle existing diseases within us. Compared to someone who doesn't have existing diseases, a person with a diagnosis spends an excessive amount of spirit to combat that diagnosis every day. This is expected to result in faster depletion of the spirit, leading to a shorter life span.

We see this every day in modern medical practice. We know that people with existing diseases, despite the availability of the best medicine, still have shorter life spans compared to those without existing disease. The shortened life span in this scenario does not manifest as rapidly as in Scenario 1, but rather, slowly progresses over a period of years. This is especially true if the disease started at a younger age.

My brother was thirty-five years old when he was diagnosed with malignant high blood pressure. This blood pressure was related to a kidney injury he had sustained as a child from an infection. During subsequent years, he was diagnosed with kidney failure, heart disease, anemia, atrial fibrillation (an abnormal rhythm of the heart), and high cholesterol levels.

Medical practitioners claimed that all these subsequent diseases are sequels to having had high blood pressure—that is true from modern medicine's perspective. He was treated for all these diseases with what modern medicine can offer. These treatments do not cure the disease, however, but control and slow the progression.

Nevertheless, his body had to continue battling those diseases 24/7. This process of constant battle required expenditure of health reserve and spirit. Over the next twenty-five years he continued fighting these diseases until, at age sixty-two, he got an infection.

At this point, he did not have enough reserve and spirit to win the battle. He died prematurely. His life was shortened. The diseases stole approximately twenty years' worth of spirit based on the average life span for a male. In contrast, both of our parents lived to be eighty-two years old.

There is a lot a person can accomplish in twenty years, but my brother was denied that opportunity. He is not alone; there are many people in his shoes. Fathers, mothers, brothers, sisters, husbands, wives, and children are going through this same process right now.

This does not mean that it's all bad news for people with diseases. It just means that relying only on modern medicine and hoping we'll be okay is not wise; eventually, we will lose the battle. Existing disease will steal our health reserve and spirit. The good news is that both health reserve and spirit can be renewed and increased depending on our actions outside of modern medicine. What we do outside of modern medicine must involve health education that focuses on real health and spirit, not fake health and disease.

Scenario 3: Slow and natural expenditure of spirit

You may know someone who has lived to be more than ninety years old without ever stepping into a hospital. Mrs. Gentle is ninety-five years old, though the average life span for an American female is only eighty years. Contrast that to the scenario above.

With the exception of childbirth, Mrs. Gentle never stepped into a hospital or took any form of medication until she was ninety years old, when she started taking medication for arthritis. She did not have many diseases diagnosed. Her spirit will be naturally spent via normal aging to a point of complete depletion until the body is not viable for the spirit's existence as we all expect in human life. Death is the only promise we have in life.

In the world of wealth and money, we speak of inflation. Inflation is the continued loss of value of the dollar year by year. For example, if you put $1,000 into a bank and left it there, in ten years the buying power of that same amount is much less than it was before.

Aging is the inflation in health. As we grow older, our spirit is spent on maintaining optimal body function, among other things (spirit is involved in several other aspects of human life). Additionally, if we have a thief (disease) stealing our health reserve and spirit, the

depletion is faster. Scenario 3 describes the effect of health inflation (aging) only, whereas Scenario 2 describes both health inflation
(aging) and the presence of a thief (disease).

From the spirit's perspective, maintenance of internal balance is
essential in all living organisms for the optimal manifestation of spirit.
Since internal balance is directly proportional to health reserve, and
subsequently health status, spirit is intricately connected to health. It
is therefore reasonable to modify our definition of health from previous chapters to the following:

> Health is human spirit's ability to withstand and
> overcome any adverse force on the body's internal
> environment. It accomplishes this by constantly
> striving to reestablish and maintain the balance
> of the internal environment at the physical, men-
> tal, emotional, and spiritual level.

CHAPTER 6

Winning View: Practical

Objectivity

Understanding human health and developing the skills to be healthy requires commitment, focus, and training. Being successful in the arena of health, as with any other aspect of life, requires a goal, a formula, and a deep understanding of the specialty. Such ambition demands focused education and training, but will in turn yield a long and vibrant life.

An objective assessment of our health education reveals that the school systems, medical systems, governments, religion, and parenting have collectively failed us. They have, in fact, disabled us, making us dependent on the very systems that let us down in the first place. These systems haven't increased our knowledge or understanding of health, nor provided the tools to be healthy. They have left us to fend for ourselves when the need arose as demonstrated during the pandemic.

I get it: not everyone wins all the time. On the other hand, everyone, without exception, can be optimally equipped to be winners.

The reality is that we have to function outside of the systems that fail us. Our lives cannot completely rely on them. This requires learning, training, and understanding the concepts of health. The best strategy is to function within the system to address disease, but function outside the system to address health. If we do that, our odds of winning increase. Functioning outside of the system implies that you have to create your own system. People who can create their own system that works in synchrony with the larger social systems are winners. This book is the first step in accomplishing a winning personal system.

In my world, most patients who need heart transplants are already at death's door, with only a couple of years left to live. Due to their weak heart, their body has changed over time. Heart disease has stolen their health reserve and spirit. Their internal environment may have initially predisposed them to heart disease, but later the environment continues to change because the disease is allowed to persist. This continuous change, in response to the disease, robs that person's spirit via rapid expenditure.

By the time they require a transplant, these patients not only need a new heart, but also a new internal environment. But no one can transplant an internal environment because the internal environment is intricately connected to the spirit, which the people must cultivate by themselves. It is the individual's responsibility.

In medicine, we give such patients a new heart and medications to ensure their body doesn't reject it. Then we send them home with regular follow-up appointments to make sure the heart is functioning well. At this point, medicine's business of caring for disease is complete. The unfortunate reality is that health has not yet been restored.

Medicine focuses on the internal environment before the transplant—to make sure that the patient can survive the surgery—but not afterwards. Post-transplant, modern medicine does not address the internal environment. The patient's internal environment is still unbalanced, not only because of the effect of prior heart disease, but also due to having a new heart. This unbalance is never addressed. It's left up to the patient, and the patient is not educated on it.

The patient returns to their pre-transplant lifestyle (which contributed to the disease in the first place), with the exception of minor changes. My experience has been that patients who create their own system to influence their internal environment win, living longer and keeping their new heart longer.

Those that did not create a new system and reverted to their pre-transplant habits lost, and did not survive as long. *Winning and losing in health has nothing to do with medicine's management of disease; it has everything to do with how we manage our own bodies.*

Rule #1: Health is a concept, not a definition.

The definition of health as described by entities like the Oxford English Dictionary, World Health Organization, media, governments, and others is not conducive to establishing or maintaining health. Those definitions favor disease care. Human health is more than what can be understood by existing definitions for health. Health has depth, dynamicity, and cumulative properties. A better and more practical way of looking at health is to think of it as a concept with a tremendous amount of information behind it. That information is currently not made available or taught by our education system or at home while growing up. Would we like to have a poorly-defined definition open to multiple interpretations, or would we like to fully understand the concept and take action? The latter seems the smarter option to me. However, based on what we have discussed so far, the following is clear.

In short, health is an ability.

It is an ability that incorporates our spirit.

Enhancing and maintaining this ability requires study of this concept.

The internal environment is the terrain that Claude Bernard argued about with Louis Pasteur. This terrain includes both the body and mind. How a person develops, increases, and maintains their ability to continuously balance their internal environment is a lifelong effort and study. The good news is we are born with this ability. It's just that we don't pay attention to it, we are not educated about it, we get distracted from it, and we lose sight of it, all while slowly losing this ability through aging (Scenario 3, Chapter 5). We lose this ability at a faster rate by consciously and unconsciously adopting a poor lifestyle, or unknowingly developing disease (Scenario 2, Chapter 5).

Rule #2: Health is a journey, not a destination.

Health is not something that we just create and move on from. Nor is it a phenomenon that completely takes care of itself throughout our life after being gifted at birth. *We* have to take care of it. Sprinters, football players, boxers, artists, actors—all of them are gifted with special abilities that they harness and execute. This special ability, however, needs to be continuously nurtured and maintained. Olympic athletes train day-in and day-out. It becomes their lifestyle. After competing, they don't stop this process; they continue training for the next competition. They retire when aging (health inflation) reduces their special abilities and no amount of training will maintain their competitive edge against younger athletes.

Health is also a journey, because an "ability" requires constant maintenance.

Good news: Health can be regularly enhanced and maintained.

Bad news: It's a lifelong process, unlike the relatively short journey of a career athlete.

Good news: We don't have to spend many hours a day to be healthy.

Bad news: Being healthy requires behavioral changes.

An athlete's competitor is the opposing athlete or team. Health's competitor is an invisible enemy—like chronic disease or a virus like COVID-19. Viruses and diseases test us. Athletes know when they're heading into competition. In health, we don't decide when the next competition is. Our invisible enemies decide.

Most often, the competition is already taking place within our bodies, and we don't even know it. We have to be prepared at all times. This information is not intended to discourage you. Being healthy is doable and actually fun, because when we start creating our own system for being healthy, we gain a vibrant and enjoyable life, as well as longevity. Our performance increases. We become more successful. And that is a win we all can live with.

Rule #3: Health is renewable.

It sounds outrageous to claim that health is renewable, but it's true because it's a component of healing that's inherent to our bodies. When end-stage heart failure patients require a heart transplant, their internal environment is severely depleted of its health reserve, and continues to decline daily. As a result, their bodies are burning their spirit at a rapid pace, and once that spirit is spent, death occurs.

When modern medicine evaluates patients for heart transplant, extensive testing is carried out. This is to ensure that their internal environment isn't severely damaged and hasn't lost its ability to regain balance with the new heart. When our internal environment is damaged to a point of no return, patients don't have enough reserve even to undergo the life-saving transplant.

If that is the case, even young patients are recommended hospice care, to spend the last of their days. Remember our previous discussion, where organs can continue to live if they are placed in a new medium of adequate spirit? In some patients, even with a new heart, the adequacy of the recipient's spirit is insufficient to function.

Fortunately, most patients are deemed to have adequate health reserve and successfully go through the surgery. These are patients that have not yet reached the point of no return in regards to their health reserve and spirit.

The expectation is that if a heart transplant is performed in time, the expenditure of health reserve and spirit (caused by the heart disease) will be terminated, and the severely damaged internal environment will slowly recover. This does, in fact, happen. As alluded to in the previous section, the rapidity and degree of rebalancing the internal environment depends on how much effort that person puts in after the transplant, outside of the medical system's recommendations.

The patients that receive a heart transplant have improved health reserve and better spirit compared to their pre-transplant status. This phenomenon suggests that health reserve and balance of the internal environment can be renewed. This is true as long as remedial measures are taken prior to our bodies reaching the point of no return, and are continued after the procedure is completed. Health is renewable—nature gave us the power to renew our health in order to survive. The responsibility of protecting and exercising that power is our own.

The final rule

Therefore, the concept of health is a lifelong adaptive behavior that confers upon our spirit the *ability* to continuously withstand and overcome any adverse force to maintain an internal balance at the physical, mental, emotional, and spiritual levels of our being, irrespective of the presence or absence of disease.

How we acquire that *ability* is our responsibility.

PART II

WHAT ELSE SHOULD I KNOW?

7 SELF-EMPOWERING CONCEPTS

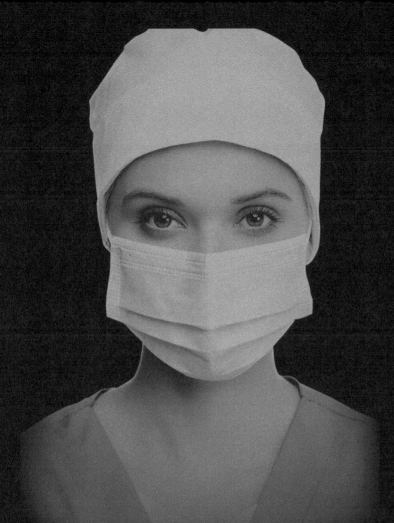

CONVERSATION
Can everyone be healthy?

CONFIRMATION
Can everyone harness
the human spirit?

CURRENCY
Can health be measured?

CHANGES
Can changes in health
be recognized?

COGNIZANCE
Can everyone become
aware of the true self?

CONTINUATION
Can everyone
renew health?

CYCLES
Can everyone be
younger and healthier?

CHAPTER 7

Conversation:
Can everyone be healthy?

The Silent Talk

Silent talk is a major contributor to winning or losing. Every human being possesses this ability, though we're not always aware of it. It controls us!

One of the most advanced skills a human possesses is the ability to communicate. We communicate in several ways—through verbal language, body language, actions, and sometimes, even through silence and inaction. All these types of conversations are carried out in two spaces. The first is between people in society—external communication. The other is within us—internal communication. The most important conversations we have are the silent communications within ourselves. In my book *Second Opinion*, it is referred to as our "internal dialogue."

This silent talk shapes our lives. In regard to success and failure, silent talk is extremely important. We listen to and trust our own silent talk much more than we rely on external communication. The silent talk places bias on what we hear from others. It clouds our ability to listen. It clouds our understanding. It masks our own spirit from fully manifesting. The silent talk has the power to engage or disengage our spirit in action.

This silent talk is our own creation, and Freud called it our super ego. The super ego is a collection of "rules of function" that we've created and have given tremendous importance. We are not born with it. As we grow older, this becomes like our parent, our teacher, our religious leader, our guide, and our peer. Why? Because these are the people that, throughout our childhood, helped create the content of this silent partner.

Our silent conversations, and the messages we receive from them, come from the silent partner within us. The content of these conversations is what we tell ourselves. We are 100 percent committed to our silent partner because we reflexively trust our silent partner—whether it leads us to success or failure. Our silent partner does not leave us when we fail, as others do, but it judges us. Whether our actions end in success or failure, we carry out the silent partner's orders like servants. These orders are silent, but let us not underestimate their power. Silent talk has the power to influence individual success or failure, because our actions are directed by it.

Have you been aware of this? Many of us are, however, most of the time, this conversation is so spontaneous that it's not in our conscious radar, and we simply carry out actions automatically. (Recommended reading: *Untethered Soul* by bestselling author Eckert Tolle, *Intention Matters* by forensic psychologist Dr. Phil, and *The Power of Intention* by motivational speaker Dr. Wayne Dyer.)

Intention is born as a product of the interaction between our silent partner and our rational brain. The silent partner, and the conversations we have with it, have the ability to break relationships, strip people of their power, push us to success or failure, and can even be the difference between life and death.

Our silent partner's default position is to urge us in the direction of "no" or negativity in order to stop us from doing something. The reason for this is that the silent partner is created by reward and punishment throughout our childhood, and punishments are more vividly embedded than rewards.

The Bad Talk

Mr. Priest was a fifty-one-year-old patient hospitalized in the cardio-vascular unit for end-stage heart failure. His heart could not pump enough blood to the rest of his body to tolerate any form of physical activity. He was on medications to "whip" the heart into pumping stronger until we could determine a plan of care. On these medications, he felt well, as long as he didn't have to move around much. He tolerated lying in bed, sitting up in a chair, and walking the short corridors of the hospital. He carried out logical conversations, and his mental function was not clouded.

His heart was failing, but fortunately, all the tests revealed that his internal environment was preserved enough to undergo heart transplant surgery. The expectation was that his internal environment would rebalance itself if we corrected the heart problem, and his life would potentially be extended by about ten to fourteen years.

With this knowledge, we recommended a heart transplant. He thought it over for a day, and then told me, "Doc, if God wants me to go, it is my time, and it looks like that is what God is telling me. I don't want a transplant."

No amount of discussion could convince him otherwise. He refused to listen to his family and friends. He even met other people who had successfully been transplanted, and still he declined. It was almost as if he had a death wish. We gave up the efforts for transplant and he died a few days later, at the age of fifty-one.

Countless examples of patients like this pass through physicians' practices—where the silent partner clouds a patient's objectivity. In this case, it appeared to end poorly, not only for the patient, but also for the patient's grieving family.

However, we don't know if it was actually a sad outcome for the patient because he lived and obeyed his silent partner. His silent partner convinced him that it was his time to pass. Most of the time, individuals do not communicate their silent conversation to outsiders. As a result, the intentions of most communications among humans are hidden. But when patients are placed in a life or death situation, they will often directly communicate the silent conversation to outsiders, just like Mr. Priest did with me. Devastatingly, there is a potential for people to misidentify their silent partner's message as coming from God.

The "Illusionist" example from Chapter 1 reveals the similarities between these two patients. Our silent partners, and the silent conversations we have with them, make us the illusionists, keeping us from objectivity.

In other words, success and failure comes from within us. A right and positive conversation within us leads to the desired outcome of that conversation by propelling us into a positive spiral. This is important if success in health is to be achieved. A negative conversation within us leads to an undesired outcome by propelling us into a downward spiral. If we have the right concept of health (as we saw in Chapter 6), and train our silent partner for the right conversation, success follows.

The Good Talk

For years, runners chased the dream of being the first to achieve a four-minute mile. Elite coaches, experts, and running enthusiasts developed several strategies and recommendations. These included: optimal weather conditions, optimal ground conditions, and the presence of a boisterous crowd to encourage the runner. Despite considering these factors, many milers continued to fail.

This failure lasted until May 6, 1954, when Roger Bannister, a twenty-five-year-old from Oxford, England, broke the barrier with a time of 3:59:40. It was on a cold day, on wet ground, and in front of only a small crowd of people—a task thought to be impossible by experts. Bannister didn't have elite training, and he ran against all the environmental recommendations. Yet, he still broke the barrier. Bannister and his silent partner confronted this task on their own. More importantly, on that day, the silent partners of several other milers changed.

Just under two months following Bannister's success, John Landy—an Australian runner—broke the record again with a time of 3:58. Within a year, three others broke the four-minute mark, and more than a thousand others have broken it over the last half-century (Taylor, 2018).

Prior to Bannister's initial success, milers were programmed to think that running a mile in under four minutes was impossible, despite consciously striving to achieve it. When Bannister broke that barrier, others started to believe that it was achievable. Their respective silent partners now believed in that possibility, and that enabled them to run a mile in under four minutes.

The Silent Partner

Our silent partner is subconsciously created throughout our childhood by the parenting we receive, the material we're taught at school, our religious teachings, and our observations of peers. As adults, that same silent partner is constantly being modified through what we learn from life experiences, the media, and whom we surround ourselves with. The silent partner consists of a collection of rules of conduct we acquire and adhere to throughout life.

Having a silent partner, and subsequently silent talk, is inevitable. What's important is to be mindful of the silent partner. It's important to resist its bias, to develop the ability to look beyond it, and objectively judge information and events independent of the silent partner.

Most of us fail in this action, due to not being mindful of it. Roger Bannister was able to judge information independently. He did not go with the mainstream recommendations. Likewise, we should be able to independently observe our silent partner. We can modify our silent partner's reasoning through retraining, and thus get rid of the old way of thinking and create a new way that better suits us.

Bannister considered all the information available to milers at the time and critically evaluated it to arrive at his own winning solution. He was the first man, ever, to break the four-minute mile barrier, and he created the possibility for others to accomplish the same. In fact, the lessons from his legacy are taught at many reputable business schools for entrepreneurial success.

Let us accept and embrace our silent partner. Having a silent partner is not a bad thing—it is inevitable. What kind of information the silent partner is composed of and what we do with our silent partner is what determines success or failure. Through training, our silent partner can help make the impossible a reality in life.

Change with the silent partner occurs under two conditions. The first is where a significant event suddenly propels us into thinking differently, like what Bannister's achievement did for the other milers' silent partners. The second is slow conditioning of the silent partner, which is what happens when we carry out repeated actions, either intentionally or unintentionally.

Unintentional training happens all around us via the circumstances we repeatedly put ourselves in, including: work, friends, co-workers, media, and other outside influences like stress. Preventing unintentional modification can be accomplished by ensuring that we always place ourselves in the right social and professional environments. In other words, by watching who and what we surround ourselves with.

Intentional training happens when we choose to change our rules of conduct via education and/or internship. The reason intentional training is required for success is because the unintentional change is already influencing our silent partner, whether we like it or not. This slow, unintentional change is what demands our conscious, intentional decisions to correct, modify, and retrain our silent partner. The default position of the silent partner is negativity arising out of fear. This is because the silent partner in us is created via the reward and punishment system we grow up with. Those who choose to intentionally cultivate a positive silent partner, win. Our environment is continuously feeding a negative silent partner because most media (social or otherwise), as well as the environment we live in, is negative. Therefore, those who do not choose to intentionally create a winning silent partner, lose.

Take for example one of my patients who illustrates this unintentional and intentional training. Mr. Addict is a young man who is a drug addict. He had befriended people that used drugs, and by placing himself in an environment of drug use, he became unintentionally addicted to drugs. He was then diagnosed with end-stage heart failure, caused by his recreational drug use.

By the time he discovered this condition, it was too late to reverse the damage, and he needed a heart transplant to save his life. However, he was not eligible due to the drug addiction. We recommended rehabilitation to treat the addiction, but he repeatedly failed the outpatient program.

After placing himself in circumstances conducive to drug addiction, his silent partner was trained to accept drug use as a coping mechanism for an underlying internal conflict. This is an example of unintentional training.

The silent partner and the silent talk were not changed by outpatient rehabilitation because he was still surrounded by his old friends. He was finally sent to a thirty-day inpatient rehab to reprogram his silent partner. This one was successful, because it took him out of the bad environment, and influenced his rational brain and silent partner without an opportunity for relapse.

Getting into a habit of drug use was the unintentional training. His addiction happened slowly and without his full awareness. The inpatient rehabilitation was intentional training to reprogram and recruit the silent partner to work with him toward success. With determination, he finally won: he reprogrammed his silent partner and received a lifesaving heart transplant. He is now a model example for our similar patients.

Neuroplasticity

Our brain is responsible for all of our "higher functions" like thinking, reasoning, logical evaluation, learning, memory, understanding, and objectivity. Through learning, the neurons (brain cells) connect and reconnect continuously to form patterns that store information in our brain. When that stored information is needed, the neurons that contain the information "light up" (become active). Collections of neurons that recall this information make up the functional unit of our memory. Our silent partner is a collection of memories that were subconsciously learned throughout our childhood. Any trigger to our brain wakes up both the area belonging to our silent partner, and the area of rational thinking—this results in communication between the two.

Changing a thinking process, and subsequently a behavior, is accomplished via a process called neuroplasticity. As stated earlier in the chapter, a trigger for change arises under two conditions: gradual change through intentional or unintentional repetition, and sudden change through impactful life events. Irrespective of the trigger, neuroplasticity underlies the process of change.

Neuroplasticity, simply put, refers to "the brain's ability to change itself" (*Psychology Today*, 2020). The brain has the ability to change existing patterns to accommodate new inputs it receives, or to compensate for lost abilities. An example of the latter is a loss of eyesight that results in heightened hearing. However, in terms of health, we're concerned with the former: accommodating new input and changing an existing pattern.

Typical examples of this plasticity include learning to drive, learning a musical instrument, or learning to play a game. These all involve repeated practice, where the brain receives new information, and then forms new circuits to store and execute the physical function. Another example, as described previously, is drug rehabilitation, where repeated reinforcement modifies the previously created addictive circuit.

I learned to drive in Sri Lanka when I was thirteen years old, and I was licensed at age seventeen. At that time, cars only had stick shift, so that's what I knew how to drive. Later, when I had to drive cars with an automatic shift, I had to intentionally retrain my brain. The ability of the brain to accommodate and change its existing neural circuitry is a very simple example of neuroplasticity.

All of us have multiple stories of neuroplasticity within us. The steps involved in this process, in medical terms, are very complicated, and beyond the scope of this book. (Recommended reading: *The Brain's Way of Healing* by Norman Doidge, MD.) Essentially, the human brain is like plastic, and like plastic, it can be molded. It becomes more difficult as we age, but it's still possible with repeated practice. The old adage, "You can't teach an old dog new tricks," does not hold true, because of our neuroplasticity.

The context of neuroplasticity is important to our discussion because the fake health system has created the wrong pattern of circuits in our brains regarding health. The current circuits in our brain are concerned with disease, which is what we've been trained to associate with health. As you read this book, the preformed "wrong" brain circuits of our silent partner are resisting our understanding and acceptance of what's being described here. This pattern of thinking has to change in order to create and maintain health, and this change can only be accomplished by reprogramming our brain.

Reprogramming requires two initial steps. First is acceptance that we currently have the wrong circuits. Second is a willingness and openness to explore other perspectives on the subject. The first step in being healthy is to realize we've been chasing the wrong idea about health. Then, we can learn the right idea and reinforce it in both our silent partner and our rational brain.

Either due to fear, ignorance, or avoidance, silent partners of most of my patients prevents them from giving health the importance it deserves in their life. If this habit is changed through education and re-training, everyone can be healthy.

CHAPTER 8

Confirmation: Can everyone harness the human spirit?

Human Spirit – The Origin of Vital-Force

There are two occasions in life where the human spirit naturally makes the biggest impact. The first impact is at the time of birth, and the second is at the time of death. The only physical difference between the two impacts is age, but they're entirely different experiences for the same individual. The impact at birth is barely recognized by an infant because an infant does not have a fully differentiated psyche. If the infant, by any chance, recognizes the impact, it is not remembered at the conscious level as an adult. None of us are aware of it. The infant is all spirit at the time of birth.

The psyche is understood in psychology (study of the psyche) as the totality of an individual's mind—including both the conscious and unconscious mind. The content of the psyche is developed over time. From a medical perspective, the psyche is the center of emotions, thoughts, and behavior. This center consciously and unconsciously mediates the body's response to the social and physical environment (dictionary.com).

Adults are able to recognize the approach of death at a conscious level because adults have a fully developed and functioning psyche.

An average American man is expected to live seventy-nine years, and a woman is expected to live eighty years. At that age, as the departure of the spirit from the human body nears, the departure is expected, often feared, and definitely felt.

Most patients requiring heart transplant only have a couple of years left to live. I have observed and discussed the feelings, wishes, and desires of countless dying people in my years of practice on different continents. The experience for both the patient and the doctor is extraordinary. One can see the spirit slowly dissipating from those ill patients. Once the threshold of no return is reached, there is no stopping that departure, irrespective of whether the body is healthy or not.

In between these two impacts, birth and death, we live our lives. During this time period, our psyche is too distracted by worldly affairs to recognize the impact of our own spirit. Nevertheless, it is important to recognize two facts. First, spirit is the source of our vital-force. Second, spirit is intricately involved in the health and survival of human beings (as we saw in Chapters 5 & 6).

The spirit is the force that gives life to our cells—it is our "vital-force." Science has not yet figured out how to identify or confirm the existence of the vital-force, nor been able to duplicate it; therefore, there's no scientific proof for the existence of spirit or vital-force.

Even though the force can't yet be described in scientific terms, that doesn't mean it's nonexistent. After all, if one had professed about the existence of nine planets in the solar system 200 years ago, people wouldn't have believed or accepted it. In 2015, astronomers have identified evidence for the existence of planet nine beyond the known planet Neptune (Witze, 2016). Whether we accept or reject the idea of spirit, the following observations are suggestive and are thought-provoking.

Spirit of Emotion

Mr. Fear, a middle-aged man, underwent heart transplant and was discharged home in stable condition. During outpatient follow-up, his wife complained that the man adamantly refused to take a shower at his own home. He was fearful of entering the bathroom. This was frustrating his wife, as it was a new habit since receiving his transplant.

Post-transplant, he was bathing daily with a sponge bath, just as he did at the hospital. Multiple conversations, investigations, and a psychiatric evaluation turned out normal—no abnormality was identified. Finally, we discovered that his transplanted heart belonged to a janitor who, while cleaning a bathroom, slipped and fell, hit his head, and died.

The recipient required multiple counseling sessions to correct the result of transference related to this habit before returning to normalcy. In modern medicine, we call this transference cell memory.

It's comforting to have a name such as "cell memory" to explain how the traumatic experience may have been transferred from the donor to the recipient. There is one problem, though. When a heart is removed from the donor's body, the nerves that are attached to the heart are cut. When that same heart is transplanted into a recipient, the nerves are not reconnected to the new heart. There is no nerve connection between the new heart and the brain of the recipient.

The big question is: how did the new heart transmit the traumatic memory to the recipient's brain? If it wasn't via the nervous system, what was it? This phenomenon has yet to be explained. Modern physicians largely ignore it, but it's gaining more attention in recent years. Scientists are beginning to use the term "energetic memory" to explain this phenomenon (Liester, 2020). Nevertheless, this unexplained and unproven phenomenon exists, just like the unexplained and unproven existence of spirit. Spirit has been considered a form of energy for a long time. It energizes the human body, enabling it to function, and it is the source of the vital-force.

Spirit of Taste

Mr. Taste, a thirty-year-old man, received a heart transplant as a life-saving measure. After transplant, he developed a craving for chicken salad. Prior to the transplant, he hated chicken salad. The patient and his family could not explain the reason for this change in taste. The donor of that patient's heart was a teenage woman who loved chicken salad. The teen had been on a diet of chicken salad for weight management at the time of her sudden death.

This phenomenon is frequently encountered in heart transplant recipients. It's unclear if other organ recipients experience the same phenomenon, like liver, kidney, and lung transplants. Traditionally, the heart is considered the seat of the soul. However, it remains a mystery whether that's the reason for heart transplant patients experiencing this phenomenon so frequently.

Spirit of Pain

Mrs. Pain, a forty-eight-year-old woman, started experiencing excruciating pain nightly after receiving a heart transplant. The pain would begin spontaneously and resolve on its own after a while. She complained of this pain during outpatient follow-up, and described it as occurring at discrete areas of the body (see illustration).

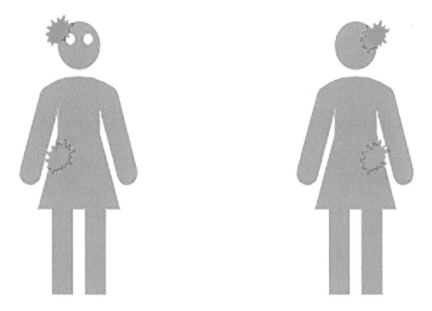

Figure 8.1: The locations of recurrent pain.

The pain typically woke her up between midnight and two a.m. We took a detailed history about this pain and worked her up with every test known to modern medicine, including a CAT scan of the head to ensure that there was no pathology in the brain. All the tests turned out normal. Review of the donor's chart revealed that the donor was a young person in their twenties who died of gunshot wounds impacting the same spots where the recipient was now complaining of pain. The reports indicated that the donor was shot at 11:59 p.m.

Spirit of Sound

Mr. Sound, a sixty-two-year-old Hispanic man underwent heart transplant. In one of the post-transplant clinic visits, his wife laughingly expressed her frustration with him. She stated that the family is no longer able to listen to Hispanic music at home, because the patient, after receiving a heart transplant, favored listening to rock and roll music, and nothing else. Apparently, the patient forbade his family from listening to any other music in the house. We later discovered that the donor of that patient's heart was a nineteen-year-old college student who liked rock and roll music, and was actively listening to it at the time of sudden death.

Spirit of Vision

Ms. Blinding, a thirty-six-year-old female heart recipient, started complaining of headaches accompanied by visions of blinding light. It would occur at any time and without any other symptoms. The transplanted heart was functioning properly. Imaging studies of the head and neurological evaluations were normal. The neurologist concluded that it was probably migraine headaches, but the patient did not have a history of migraine headaches prior to transplant. The patient was very distraught by these symptoms and was disabled during these attacks. She described the experience as if she was almost paralyzed during her headaches. We were at a loss.

Review of this patient's donor chart revealed that the heart donor was a young individual who died of a head-on motor vehicle collision at nighttime. The donor was an unrestrained passenger in the front seat. During the collision, the donor was ejected from the vehicle and died of head trauma. The blinding light and headaches can be associated with the donor's time of death, and it can be an explanation for the symptoms that the recipient was experiencing. The transplanted heart could have carried the last memory of the donor as cell memory.

Every post-heart transplant patient undergoes a procedure called a heart biopsy to confirm that the body isn't rejecting the transplanted heart. The procedure starts by making a needle puncture in the neck and accessing the neck vein. An instrument called a bioptome is passed through the vein, and it takes very small pieces of the heart to investigate under the microscope. During this procedure, the patient's heart rate, blood pressure, and oxygen levels (called the vital signs) are continuously monitored. The procedure takes about thirty to forty minutes to complete.

During one such procedure, Ms. Blinding became unresponsive. Multiple attempts from my physician-colleague (who was preforming the procedure) to communicate with the patient failed. The patient was not under sedation and there was no seizure activity. Her vital signs were all normal and unchanged, even though the patient was not responsive. Within a couple of minutes, the patient regained responsiveness.

She then stated that she'd been experiencing bright lights in her vision and was unable to communicate, even though she was able to hear when my colleague was trying to arouse her. Medically, my colleague, who is a trained and board-certified heart failure specialist, could not explain what happened to the patient. The patient also could not explain it. This is the first incident, to the best of my knowledge, where a patient being medically monitored without sedation experienced this phenomenon, and modern medicine cannot explain it.

The Might of an Aligned Spirit

This is a tale of two patients who used their spirit in their own way, leading to two completely different outcomes. Mr. Denial is a forty-four-year-old man with end-stage heart failure. Ms. Sunshine is an eighty-year-old woman with the same condition. Their medical diagnoses were identical. Both of them, at the time of referral, were recommended the next level of therapy for their condition in order to extend their lives.

Mr. Denial refused to adjust his lifestyle to suit the degree of illness. He was fearful and anxious. Usually, this kind of disengagement happens through denial from the silent partner. His intense emotions prevented his spirit from aligning with the situation. In other words, his spirit was not given a chance to engage and manifest—he did not recruit the spirit. By not changing his lifestyle, he was not renewing his vital-force, either. He totally relied on his emotions for survival while his vital-force was slowly depleted.

Finally, he became aware of his approaching death and wanted to do everything to survive, including advanced therapies. But, by that point, it was too late: he was bed-bound, and his condition had deteriorated his health too much. Attempts to provide supportive care failed, and he subsequently died.

His death was not a failure of modern medicine, however. Unfortunately, his health reserve and vital-force had been depleted to a point of no return, and no marvel of modern medicine could regenerate that vital-force. Regeneration of vital- force is entirely dependent on the individual. If a disease is already present, timing is everything.

Ms. Sunshine, on the other hand, was very engaged. Her face lit up at the suggestion that there may be a pathway to prolong her life. Her emotions did not cloud her, and she asked, "What do I have to do?" Her silent partner was recruited. The strength and alignment of the spirit was clear. At the time of our interaction, she was frail. We did not think that she would survive the major surgery at age eighty.

She went home and worked to renew her health reserve by undergoing regular physical rehabilitation. When ready, she underwent major heart surgery, where a mechanical circulatory support device was placed to help her heart pump. Today, she continues to exhibit her spirit and allow the spirit to fuel her life.

The involvement of the spirit in health and survival cannot be underestimated. It can be the difference between life and death, and is the same in other aspects of life. Success, even in the sectors of work, finances, entrepreneurship, and relationships, is dependent on the alignment and involvement of our spirit. Even though this patient was eighty years old, the strength of her spirit successfully carried her old body through the major surgery. The might of the spirit made the difference.

This chapter is written in a contextual form to exhibit the importance of the spirit and the force generated from it (vital-force) in the realm of health and survival. Modern medicine and modern thinking do not acknowledge the human spirit's involvement in that realm. The obvious reason for this is that spirit is still an abstract concept and scientists have not discovered proof of it.

Yet every single one of us is aware of our mighty spirit, its power, and its energy, although we ignore it. The observations described above are thought-provoking and strengthen our understanding of spirit. They illustrate the spirit's ability to perform in ways that still cannot be explained by science, just as we have no explanation for the cell memory of a transplanted organ to communicate with the recipient's brain.

People, who have been successful in any undertaking, including health, are those that have recognized the presence and power of the spirit. These are the winners, and engaging the spirit is the secret to winning. Those that fail have not yet learned how to engage the spirit to influence outcomes in their life. They have not recognized the secret. Those whose spirits align with anything they do are happy and content in what they do. Those with non-aligned spirits are miserable and unhappy. What group would we like to belong to?

The power of the spirit is limitless. It can be harnessed for success. One just has to learn how. At this point, it's sufficient to attest that patients who engaged their spirit survived, despite being in poor health, while those that did not engage their spirit perished, even with good physical health.

CHAPTER 9

Currency: Can health be measured?

The Known

The word "currency" brings money to mind. Money is the currency of wealth. For most people, personal success revolves around the accumulation of wealth, estimated as a person's "net worth." This net worth is expressed in the respective country's currency. The well-known idiom, "Keeping up with the Joneses," refers to showing off that we have more money than our neighbor.

We work for money. We build businesses and companies that make money. If we don't own companies or businesses, we invest in other people's companies through stocks to increase our own money. Money brings people together. Money divides people. Money consumes people's time. Our children spend their entire childhood preparing to make money as employees. We spend our entire youth saving money for retirement. When we become employees, we sell a good chunk of our life in exchange for money in the form of time. We sell our time for a minimum price of $11.00 an hour in Arizona, the state's minimum wage. Governments and states decide how much our time is worth, and we let them. Governments print and circulate money. That's how powerful the currency of wealth is in our life. We don't question the true nature of it.

Money has power, and yet it has no real value. Money is a medium by which wealth is traded. Wealth is comprised of possessions of value. A quantifiable medium is needed for anything to be valued, measured, and expressed. Money is the currency in which the value of our possessions are estimated and traded. Everyone, even children, know of money.

In the old days, trading was done via articles of possession such as livestock, spices, precious metals, etc. Later, governments created paper money. Even later, paper money became plastic with the use of credit cards. One can carry a plastic credit card and exchange money without ever touching physical money. In the current era, most of us don't even see or feel money—it's all exchanged through electronics as mere digital numbers.

A lot of people don't even carry money anymore, but even so they carry the concept of money. That concept is so strong that the tangible medium of wealth no longer has to be tangible for us to believe in it. We believe in a financial abstract. Because money is tangible, we continue to deal with it.

How about our abstract concept of health?

The Unknown

Health and wealth are intricately linked, as evidenced by their simultaneous collapse during the pandemic. But unlike wealth, health differs in regard to measurability. One of the reasons we don't pay attention to health is because health does not have an accepted, tangible currency for quantification. What we cannot estimate or assess, we tend to ignore.

The human mind gravitates toward aspects of life that can be perceived by our five senses. That which can be perceived by the senses, appears more real to us. Tangibility becomes a strong driving force in our gravitation toward any pursuit. That which is not quantifiable becomes less consequential by comparison. That is, in the case of health, until we lose it and become ill.

When seemingly healthy people contracted COVID-19, they suddenly realized that they weren't healthy. They feared death. There was still no clear concept of what was lost, but everyone called it health. Because disease is tangible (in the form of symptoms), and health is abstract, we focus on what is tangible—disease. But, in real life, diseases are not the only cause of loss of vital-force. For example, aging slowly depletes our vital-force. Unhealthy behaviors deplete our vital-force. Still, the amount of health lost remains immeasurable due to the absence of a known medium for quantification.

Our understanding of health in the example of COVID-19 is in sharp contrast to what happens in wealth. Take, for example, the economic crisis, which resulted from the pandemic. Millions of people became jobless, even if they did not catch the virus. Their livelihoods were lost, and some lost their homes and businesses. This time, the threat to life was not due to disease, but due to loss of wealth. But unlike health, we are actually able to calculate how much money a person lost during the economic crisis. We do not hear or see any mention of measurability of true health without mention of disease either in the media, health system, or government. Yet it is, after all, the fear of losing our health that collapsed the economy. Fear, cannot be measured. Anything that cannot be quantified can be manipulated.

The reason health is ignored, and the system's efforts to develop a vaccine are maximized, is because the entire understanding of this health crisis has been carried out within health systems that provide disease care—not healthcare. The medical system is concerned with disease. For you and me, it should be about understanding health outside of disease leading to not only creating a vaccine but also enhancing the underlying health status of people. Existing systems in most countries fail in this aspect. While this is bad news from population perspective, it gives us an opportunity, as individuals, to create a personal health system of our own.

We have to face it; the winners in both the health and economic crisis of COVID-19 are those that did not have to rely on the government and the health system. Actually, governments and health systems abandoned countless people, and were able to take care of only those that had the disease from a health crisis perspective (and even then, not everyone received care). Even if we wanted to rely on these systems for our own health, it would be a major let down and argues for supplementing with our own system as well.

Health is an important possession. Despite this, we take it for granted, and realize its value only once we've lost it. As such, it's more advantageous to recognize that precious possession when we actually possess it, rather than discovering it after it's lost. Any possession has value, and value needs a medium for measurement and expression. Health, therefore, needs a medium—a currency—for us to be able to align with health without disease being part of it.

The Idea

Observing the suffering that patients go through when health is diminished reveals an important finding: not all patients suffer at the same level because not all diseases rob us of health to the same degree. There is gradation, like shades of a color, indicating levels of health gain and health loss, which can then be measured.

Even though I am a practicing physician, this aspect of health was not apparent for a long time, because it's not the focus of medical practice. After almost thirty-five years of observing dying patients and exploring health and disease, it dawned on me that health should be measurable—we just have not identified the currency of health. If we did, being healthy would be achievable for more than just a few.

The most successful interventions in health are achieved under three conditions. First, a patient must have a goal, or what I like to call a "finish line." Second, they must accept that a change in their silent partner is needed to achieve that goal. Third, there must be an action with measurable results to convince them of their daily progress. In short, health interventions require a goal, a realization, and an action. The goal and action involves measurability. The measurable progress achieved provides motivation to continue to change the silent partner.

A determination to achieve a goal without measurable action, or taking action without a goal, will not lead to success. This rule is true in any aspect of life. Mr. Lazy is a perfect example of this phenomenon in health.

Mr. Lazy was debilitated and had end-stage heart failure. He required a heart transplant, but was not a candidate because he lacked the motivation and enthusiasm. He needed to physically and nutritionally improve, but he couldn't mount the effort to rehabilitate his body enough to safely undergo transplant surgery. Additionally, he needed to comply with medical recommendations. He was simply being a slug, and he was fast-approaching death despite the effort and encouragement of the medical team.

At every visit, Mr. Lazy came to the clinic in a wheelchair with swollen legs and a depressed attitude. We emphasized to him the importance of compliance, physical rehabilitation, and nutritional resuscitation, but every time we confronted him, he (his silent partner) had an excuse for not being compliant or enthusiastic.

Then, one of his clinic visits was life-changing.

We sat down and had a heart-to-heart discussion about his heart disease (no pun intended), what it meant for his life, and how he was nearing death. We firmly informed him of the need to get stronger, walk to the clinic without a wheelchair, and show adherence to recommendations. He was told that failure to achieve these goals would mean that he was going to die.

That clinic visit was different for Mr. Lazy. He listened intently and gave no excuses for his failure. He looked me in the eye and said, "Doc, I am going to do it." That was it. He meant what he said, and said nothing more.

A month later, I ran into him in the hospital, and almost didn't recognize him. He appeared about ten years younger, had no leg swelling, and most importantly, he was not in a wheelchair. He was a different man. He walked all on his own and was in a happy, upbeat mood. He'd been going to cardiac rehab regularly, maintaining compliance with diet and medications, and was working closely with the medical team. Later, he was accepted for evaluation to undergo heart transplant.

This is an example of the modification of negative silent talk into positive silent talk, achieved through the process of neuroplasticity. Specifically, Mr. Lazy needed a goal to achieve, guidance on the measurability of his condition to monitor progress, and a heartfelt discussion that clearly illustrated his barriers for achieving his goal. When measurability became possible through a clearly-defined goal, personal success followed.

The Currency

Health, as we have learned so far, is an ability to overcome adverse forces on our physical, mental, emotional, and spiritual balance. The tools we possess to carry out that ability are our physical bodies and our minds. Cells in our body remain ready to overcome adversity by maintaining the optimal balance of our body's internal environment. The drive for overcoming the adverse forces is the instinct for survival. The source of this instinct is our spirit. The fuel for continuously supporting and promoting the optimal balance is the vital-force. Our spirit constantly provides the vital-force that feeds the body's cells to maintain optimal balance, and thus, allows us to overcome any adversity to our self.

If an adverse agent, like the coronavirus, is able to get a foothold in our system, the vital-force draws from its reserve to fight, overcome, and eliminate the adverse agent, which rebalances our internal environment. *The ability to generate a vital-force is what makes us healthy.* This engagement of the spirit is dynamic and constant, and it never stops until we die. *The spirit's vital-force manifests as energy.*

As with any form of energy, the vital-force is intangible. Take electricity for example. Electricity itself is intangible, but its effects are perceptible and measurable. We can see the light produced by a bulb, feel the air moved by a fan, and recognize a moving car. If there is no electricity, our cell phones, computers, and fridges won't operate.

The spirit's energy, or "vital-force," is similar. It isn't tangible, but its effects are perceivable. All healthcare workers witness the effects of spirit and the vital-force every time they care for a patient. Yet we take it for granted and ignore it because it's not quantifiable. The energy generated by our spirit is the vital-force, and the constant flow of this vital-force through our body and mind is the "life-flow."

The vital-force flows constantly to provide the fuel to sustain life, thereby fulfilling the survival instinct. When this life-flow stops, we die, just like companies and people go bankrupt when their cash flow stops. The vital-force is to health what money is to wealth. *Vital-force is the currency of health, and life-flow is to health as cash flow is to wealth.* Just like how cash flow is important in building wealth, life-flow is key in building health.

The concept of vital-force flowing through our body to sustain us is not new—it's been around for thousands of years. Several terms exist to describe this vital-force in different civilizations, cultures, religions, and philosophies. Perhaps the most commonly used and easily understood term is "spirit."

Experiments to understand the spirit have failed, and therefore, there is no clear concept of spirit in modern medical practice. As it stands currently, the understanding is confined to our belief that death occurs when the spirit leaves the body.

The Ayurvedic tradition of the Hindus referred to this energy as "prana," and it flows through the body and is stored in centers called "chakras." Traditional Chinese medicine refers to this energy as "Qi" (pronounced Chi), and it flows through distinct acupuncture channels. Scientology refers to it as "thetan." Ancient Greeks called it "pneuma." Galvani called it "animal electricity." Paracelsus called it "quintessence." In homeopathy, it is called the "vital-force." In anthropology and theosophy, it is called the "health aura."

Once the currency of health as energy is understood, conceptualizing health becomes a little easier. The amount of vital-force available at any given time determines our status of health. Just as currency enables us to quantify wealth, the concept of vital-force brings us closer to a similar understanding of health.

The amount of vital-force determines the strength or weakness of our terrain and its ability to ward off adverse forces in our body, as Claude Bernard conceptualized it. The stronger the vital-force, the stronger the terrain becomes, and the stronger our ability to overcome adverse forces. A strong vital-force thus means our bodies are less susceptible to diseases like COVID-19, or to other chronic diseases. Winning and losing in health depends on the battle between our vital-force and the adverse forces.

The next step in the context of health is to determine its gradations so that we can monitor the status of our health. If the status of health can be regularly monitored, we do not need to wait for the appearance of disease to identify a reduction in health.

CHAPTER 10

Changes: Can changes in health be recognized?

Up and Down

Health, as we have discovered, is an *ability* of ours, and therefore, it's a dynamic process. This ability refers to the degree we can continue to maintain the internal balance of our body in the face of adverse forces. Whether this adverse force is external (e.g. COVID-19) or internal (e.g. extreme anxiety and depression) does not matter. The components that are instrumental in maintaining a healthy balance—including our cells, the vital-force, and life-flow (the speed of vital-force generation or depletion)—must be constantly engaged in a dynamic state. The generation of vital-force is "positive life-flow," and the depletion of vital-force is "negative life-flow." This is similar to positive and negative cash flow in finances. Positive and negative life-flow is constantly in flux, moving up and down. Winning and losing in health depends on the ratio of positive and negative life-flow.

We are all born with a healthy and functioning internal environment, and adequate vital-force to maintain the healthy balance of that environment. You may be wondering: what about children born with congenital abnormalities and birth defects? Even children with birth defects are born with adequate spirit, but they have altered physical functioning. Birth defects result from the influence of the parental spirit and genetics. In these children, the abnormal function may drain their vital-force at a faster rate. This leads to a shorter life span compared to an individual with normal physical function. This is similar to driving a car with unequal tire pressure resulting in accelerated fuel burn and a shorter driving distance. Corrective surgeries can repair some of these birth defects and normalize their function to a degree. This repair reduces the draining of vital-force/life-flow, and extends their life.

We're exposed to both internal and external factors that influence our vital- force on a daily basis. This influence can either be favorable or adverse toward our vital-force, though the collective sum of these influences is adverse in nature—meaning, vital-force is depleted more than it's generated on a daily basis. This is because we live in a society that takes more from us than it gives.

These influences disrupt the internal balance inside our body, and tip the balance one way or the other. When our internal balance is disrupted, the vital-force is engaged to rebalance it. This results in expenditure of some of the vital-force, and that energy needs to be replaced in order to return to its original balance. The replacement of vital-force is carried out by borrowing energy from our spirit, or by regenerating it. The human body is naturally designed this way—the law of nature governs the function of all that is part of it.

Consider Mr. Rich and his financial practices as an illustration. Mr. Rich has a savings account and several checking accounts to his name. One of his checking accounts is specifically for health-related expenses. The savings account is for general support of all other aspects of his life, such as education, travel, entertainment, food, etc., but most importantly, his retirement. A portion of the money from his savings account is allocated to the health-related checking account. He also has overdraft protection linking the health-related checking account and the savings account. There is a debit card associated with his health-related checking account.

One day, Mr. Rich finds he's run out of toiletries. This event presents an imbalance in his busy, daily routine. He simply goes to a store, purchases these articles, and pays with his debit card. His immediate life is rebalanced.

However, the checking account now has less money, resulting in an imbalance of its own. This imbalance can be fixed in two ways. One is for Mr. Rich to generate that amount of money and deposit it into his checking account. Another is to simply borrow that amount of money from the savings account and deposit it into the health-related checking account. What's more, he also has overdraft protection. Even if he does not actively transfer that money from his savings, the bank will automatically handle the transfer when the balance in the checking account falls below a certain amount. If the bank did this through overdraft protection, Mr. Rich would not even know about it until he checks the bank's balance sheet (that is, if he's in the habit of regularly checking the balance sheet).

The process of maintaining balance in health is similar. The savings account is our spirit. The health-related checking account, and the money within it, is the vital-force allocated by the spirit for our health. At any given time, all of these components are in balance. In the example, running out of sanitary supplies is the adverse force. Being able to immediately purchase them with existing money from the health-related checking account compares in health to using existing vital-force to rebalance the cells.

Once the purchase is complete, Mr. Rich's imbalance is corrected. Similarly, once the cells rebalance, our body's internal imbalance is corrected but an imbalance of vital-force is created, which requires rebalancing of its own. Renewing the vital-force through healthy behavior is similar to Mr. Rich earning the amount of money to replace what he spent, whereas replacing his money by transferring from his savings account is like taking more out of our spirit and thus depleting the spirit's reserve.

A transfer carried out via overdraft protection may not even appear on Mr. Rich's radar on a daily basis. It is the same in health. Unless we make a conscious daily effort to pay attention to the fluctuations in our health status, the ups and downs of our health will remain unknown to us. That is, until a disease strikes, and we find out that we've lost not just the vital-force reserve, but also part of the spirit.

When the savings account is empty, Mr. Rich's financial system goes into chaotic disbalance, and he becomes bankrupt. Likewise, when the spirit is all spent, the human body goes into a chaotic disbalance and dies. This has been evident in my practice with hospitalized and non-hospitalized patients on multiple occasions. When a patient's spirit is spent, they do not survive, no matter how advanced the medical care is.

The HIDE Quadrants

Disease can progress within us undetected and be invisible. Disease causes a disbalance of our internal environment. However, a disease to develop, our internal environment, the terrain, should have already been altered with regard to its balanced state. Alteration in the state of balance can happen to different degrees. The degree of imbalance depends on the ratio between vital-force generation and depletion. As discussed previously, adverse forces can begin to slowly shift the balance between vital-force generation and depletion leading to alteration in the overall balance of our internal environment. This imbalance predisposes to disease development. When disease develops, it becomes an additional adverse force, further shifting the internal balance negatively. As a result, the state of balance at any given time can be placed into four different quadrants based on the degree of shift in overall balance.

These quadrants describe the ratio resulting from vital-force generation (positive life-flow) and vital- force depletion (negative life-flow). What quadrant the state of balance falls into depends on several factors: the degree and continuity of adverse force, the degree of effort we put into eliminating the adverse force, and the degree of vital-force available for this purpose. Generation of vital-force depends on what we actively do, while depletion of vital-force depends on how strong and how many adverse forces are active. The following figure depicts the four quadrants of our internal balance.

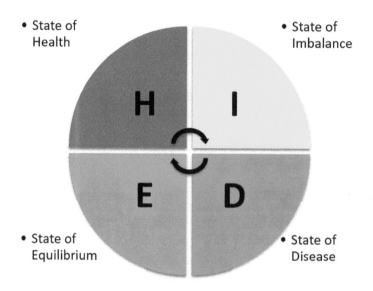

Figure 10.1: The HIDE quadrants.

During the 2020 pandemic, everyone neglected to focus on how the status of different people's health (terrain) handled the infection (adverse force). We now know that health is our ability to engage the three components that collectively provide us this ability. Namely, the internal balance of the cells, the vital-force that energizes and executes this balance, and the spirit that supplies the vital-force. *The only way for us to influence our spirit and the balance is through influencing vital- force generation and depletion (Figure 10.2).* The government and the misdirected health system were so intensely focused on disease that it blinded them to those who survived the infection.

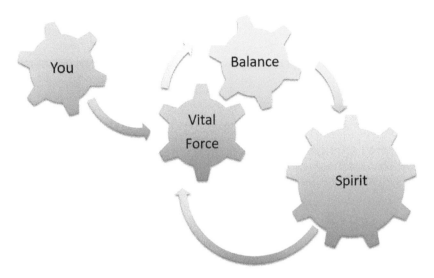

Figure 10.2: The three determinants of health and our point of influence.

A State of Health – The "H" Quadrant

People in this quadrant are in a state of good health. This is the state where the balance of the internal environment is optimal—where the body has the best ability to ward off adverse forces. In this state, the rate of vital-force generation far exceeds the rate of vital-force depletion.

The people belonging to Group 2, as mentioned in Chapter 2, had this optimal balance of their internal environment. They were able to win the battle against COVID-19 unscathed. Even though the balance is always in flux, the people in this state can quickly mount a resistance and overcome adverse force due to their ability to recruit enough vital-force to support their cells' effort to rebalance.

This ability to rapidly deploy a response is the "health reserve" discussed in Chapter 2. The aim of an evidently healthy person is to achieve and maintain this state of balance. In this state, no diagnosis of disease exists. A doctor cannot identify any physical abnormalities. People maintaining this level of optimal balance are referred to as being asymptomatic.

Ms. Runner is one of the younger staff members who worked with my team throughout the pandemic. All of our office staff was tested when acute testing for COVID-19 became available. The only person who tested positive was Ms. Runner, who had no symptoms whatsoever. She is an example of those in the "H" quadrant, and she falls within the group of people who didn't even know they had contracted the virus.

The silent partner of people in this quadrant is working along-side their will to be healthy. When we're young, being healthy comes with ease because we have plenty of vital-force and spirit. For older adults, it's harder, and it requires prioritization and effort. It becomes even harder with the added stress of responsibilities like work and family. This is why being healthy is a continuous effort. The decision to focus on and prioritize health by these individuals is supported by their silent partner. Their silent partner aligns with the decision to prioritize health, and they do whatever is necessary to maintain it. Such alignment and commitment is the first step of a continuous effort. Can you say the same about yourself? Unless our silent partner truly partners with us, no success can be achieved.

Belonging to this quadrant is like being ultra-rich, with a vast retirement fund and smartly-diversified portfolio. This reflects our description of Mr. Rich, who understands how money "works" and manages it well to create personal wealth. His income far exceeds his expenses. We want to do the same in health: understand how it works, learn the principles, and develop a system to create adequate reserves of vital-force to preserve personal health.

A State of Imbalance – The "I" Quadrant

As our internal balance begins to shift away from a healthy state, we move from "H" quadrant into this quadrant. This is a state in which our body is constantly behind in its balancing effort. It's fervently trying to regain balance, but is prevented from doing so due to a lack of adequate vital-force, lack of personal effort, or a persistent and strong adverse force. In this state, vital-force generation barely matches vital-force depletion by an adverse force.

An example of a persistent adverse force is chronic stress. Chronic stress causes a constant imbalance of our internal environment. Stress, either real or perceived, elicits fight or flight reaction that leads to biological changes in our body. When the stress is perpetuated, it becomes chronic. As a result, the biological reaction is also perpetuated and leads to development of generalized inflammation in the body. Persistent inflammatory state predisposes our body to be susceptible to development of diseases (Segerstrom, 2004). Our internal environment is constantly trying to correct the state of inflammation and thus depletes vital-force leading to an overall imbalance. The imbalance persists until the stress is eliminated. Other examples of such adverse forces include: burnout, chronic sleep deprivation, chronic consumption of unhealthy diet, and persistent grief, anger, and depression to name a few.

At this level of imbalance, people do not feel the symptoms of disease, because a disease has not yet resulted. What they feel is minor episodic symptoms, such as tiredness, fatigue, slowness of their mental faculties, lack of motivation, subtle depression, occasional headaches, indigestion, abdominal bloating, minor aches and pains, etc.

If we go to the doctor in this state, they probably won't find anything wrong with us. The physical exam and laboratory testing will be within normal range. This is because, at this point, the problem is only a subtle internal energetic imbalance. A disease will not have been diagnosed, but physicians may suspect one is present in its initial, undetectable state.

People in this quadrant are those we discussed as belonging to Group 3 in Chapter 2. These are people who were infected with coronavirus, developed mild symptoms, and improved without requiring hospitalization. They were healthy enough to overcome the additional imbalance the virus caused. They still had adequate vital-force to rebalance themselves to the state prior to infection. Even after beating the virus, this group does not shift back into the "H" quadrant, unless they also eliminate the persistent adverse force that placed them in the "I" quadrant to begin with.

During the pandemic this group of people are those that developed minor symptoms and later struggled to completely get rid of those minor symptoms and went on to develop what we now call "post COVID-19 syndrome" compared to those that completely recovered. This late sequel of the syndrome is characterized by mild ongoing symptoms of COVID-19 that persist months after the acute infection is identified (www.cdc.gov).

Even though these two sects were in the same "I" quadrant, they were at different levels of internal balance as depicted in Figure 10.3. Those that completely recovered were closer to "H" quadrant as opposed to those that developed the post COVID-19 syndrome.

The silent partner of people in this quadrant continues to pay attention to other priorities in life, and places their health-related efforts on the back burner. The people in this group don't take any effort in renewing health, either due to poor prioritization or due to an illusion of being healthy. These people are on their way to developing disease.

Belonging to this quadrant is like Mr. Pretender, who is a middle-class employee, with a big house, expensive cars, and luxury vacations—someone who appears rich to the outside world. Except, he's actually living paycheck to paycheck, always trying to keep up with the demand on a daily basis to maintain the illusion of a rich life. His income is equal to his expenses. Any slight perturbation, like an unexpected expense, could cripple his life, resulting in a major setback.

It's important to recognize when we're in this "I" quadrant because, if allowed to be in it too long, we will become more and more susceptible to developing disease. Once disease develops, we move into the next quadrant, "D", where the imbalance worsens. Identifying the insult that causes a shift from quadrant "H" to "I" allows us to take the necessary action to shift back into "H", preventing the development of disease.

Whether we shift back into the "H" quadrant or continue to progress into the "D" quadrant is a matter of time. If we spend too long in the "I" quadrant, our vital-force continues to deplete, and disease follows. If we recognize this depletion and quickly take corrective action, we have the potential to shift back to the "H" quadrant.

A State of Disease – The "D" Quadrant

This is a state where the internal harmony of our cells and organs is in significant disbalance. In this state, vital-force depletion far exceeds our vital-force generation. Finding ourselves in this quadrant indicates that we've either failed to recognize the transition into the "I" quadrant, or we did nothing to shift back into the "H" quadrant after transitioning into the "I" quadrant. The adverse force has gained so much strength within us that the vital-force's effort to regain balance is always behind. At this level, disease manifests. We have already failed our health.

At this point, the question is whether we give up and allow the disease to overcome us, or we generate enough will power to shift into a new rebalanced state—the "E" quadrant. Will power is a manifestation of the strength of our spirit. When a disease has been present for a long time in a person and has depleted their spirit, they lose the will to live.

It is easy to find ourselves in the "D" quadrant. This is the quadrant that modern medicine excels in. We develop symptoms and signs of a disease—the invisible enemy manifests. Rapidly-developing infections such as COVID-19 are not the only threats we face, however. Even chronic diseases like diabetes, high blood pressure, emphysema, chronic kidney disease, arthritis, depression, and anxiety are also invisible enemies. These chronic diseases start at a stage when we're in the "I" quadrant and believe we are healthy—the state of illusion we discussed in Chapter 1. Some people continue that illusion, remaining in denial even when they are obviously sick and hospitalized.

Science has shown that the early stages of atherosclerosis of our blood vessels (a condition that predisposes the person to future heart attacks and strokes) is present in children as young as ten years old. And yet, heart attacks most frequently occur in people aged forty to eighty years.

This illustrates how long a chronic adverse force can be present in our body before symptoms manifest. In this case, the ages between ten and forty represent the time we spend in the "I" quadrant, not knowing of the ongoing battle within ourselves. This is the time that most young people are under the illusion that they are healthy, where they typically live the most toxic-lifestyle, calling it "enjoying their youth." This is the time when we excessively spend our vital-force. It's no wonder why even young people succumbed to COVID-19. They'd drained their checking account and were unwittingly living off of what remained in their savings.

In the "D" quadrant, the disease is in the process of overwhelming the person's vital-force. It disbalances the harmony of their internal environment. The cells in the body, having been left uncorrected in the imbalanced state ("I" quadrant) for too long, have changed their structure and behavior in order to adapt to the chronic toxic insult and begin to exhibit unhealthy function—this is like surrendering to the enemy and accepting new rules of function.

These changes may be related to one organ, several organs, or generalized (like a disease of the immune system) depending on the predisposition of the person. The changes in cell behavior are what produce the symptoms we experience, and the changes in structure and function are what doctors look for in blood tests and imaging studies like X-rays, CAT, ultrasound, and MRI scans.

Once the enemy is given a diagnosis, doctors can treat it with medications to weaken the disease, thereby slowing the depletion of vital-force. Medications are prescribed if the disease is at a stage when there are only functional (not structural) changes of cells and organs. If there are structural changes, medications may not be enough, and doctors must perform surgery to either correct the faulty structure or completely remove it.

In this quadrant, the physicians' efforts are to support the body to sustain and tolerate the disease. If we have more than one of the same type of organ, and one is faulty, we can remove it. If the disease is too overwhelming, repair of the damaged organ may not be enough. In these instances, the organ needs to be replaced, and we call this process organ transplantation. Heart, kidneys, liver, lungs, pancreas, intestines, and many other areas of the body can be transplanted.

All efforts of modern medicine are supportive in nature. Most patients believe that the supportive care will take care of the disease entirely, and then they can return to their old habits—this is where they are mistaken. First, supportive care neither eliminates disease, nor does it completely overwhelm disease. Remember: medications and surgeries are control measures. They only slow the depletion of vital-force by the disease. This means that the patient must put in the effort to improve vital-force generation.

Most patients fail to recognize this, and subsequently fail themselves in life. The point here is: modern medicine's supportive measures are tools to curb only the disease. Regaining our internal balance and shifting into the "I" or "E" (described below) quadrant, and then possibly into the "H" quadrant has to originate internally from within us.

The tools to execute this shift are under our control, and they include: our silent partner, our cells, our vital-force, and our spirit. We have to strengthen and engage these rebalancing tools in conjunction with the disease-weakening tools (medication, surgery) provided by modern medicine (example of Mr. Artist in Chapter 3). Patients who continue to decline are those that don't engage these personal tools. Patients who engage their own tools and change their behavior become winners against disease.

The silent partner of people who fall in this quadrant has either not aligned with being healthy, or is in denial. Until the silent partner changes its attitude, there will be no progress. Remember Mr. Lazy? He needed a heart-to-heart talk for his silent partner to realize that without change, there is no winning. Until that change happened, he was failing. Once the silent partner committed to overcoming the disease, everything changed. His ability to execute what was required for generation of vital-force increased.

Remember: health is an ability.

Looking back to Mr. Pretender, he is not just living paycheck-to-paycheck anymore. His financial debt is now greater than what he makes. Consider a situation where he is actively borrowing, but paying nothing back—he'll continue to accumulate debt, and soon go bankrupt. The borrowing of money in this case is similar to us taking medications to supplement the rebalancing process in health. Any small event that further disbalances Mr. Pretender's situation can result in bankruptcy. In regards to health, this represents hospitalizations and even death.

Almost all of my patients are like Mr. Pretender in regards to their health—in the "D" quadrant. Most of them, unfortunately, are not given the information contained in this book. Why? The information in this book cannot be passed along in a twenty-minute doctor's visit. Health education and knowledge is the patient's responsibility, but no one is teaching that. Doctors are too busy prescribing medications and performing surgeries, trying to keep their patients afloat.

A State of Equilibrium – The "E" Quadrant

Being in this quadrant means that we are getting better—either healing from an acute disease or improving from the exacerbation of an existing chronic one. Either way, being in this quadrant means that a few events have taken place. First and foremost, the individual made a commitment to address their health (in addition to disease) with the support of their silent partner. Second, the silent partner is being retrained through neuroplasticity (this is what Mr. Lazy did by engaging in regular physical and nutritional rehabilitation after committing to beat the disease). As a result of these efforts, vital-force generation has increased, while medications and other supportive efforts are simultaneously decreasing vital-force depletion. A new equilibrium is being established.

The "E" quadrant is where tremendous self-effort is carried out to change the generation-to-depletion ratio. Every person who leaves a hospital is in this quadrant at the time of discharge. However, their continued improvement depends upon further effort by the patient.

Once a disease initiates the course of disbalance, the only way to change that course is to reverse the ratio of vital-force generation-to-depletion. Medications and surgeries will decrease the vital-force depletion, but the question is, are we doing our part to increase vital-force generation?

This is the situation of Group 4 described in Chapter 2, those patients who were hospitalized with COVID-19 and survived.

During the hospitalization, their vital-force depletion was minimized by the supportive care provided by modern medicine. Concurrently, their spirit was directing vital-force toward a new balance. In this state, the rate of vital-force depletion was actively decreasing while the rate of vital-force generation was increasing, moving toward a new equilibrium.

Once a disease develops, it's hard to achieve an optimal balance like in the "H" quadrant. Nevertheless, a rebalanced state can be achieved that gets us closer to the balance that exists in "H" quadrant. Accomplishing and remaining in a rebalanced state requires constant effort by the individual. This is the predicament most of my patients find themselves in, but they fail due to a lack of awareness of being in this quadrant. As a result, the disease continues to progress, resulting in re-hospitalization and further decline.

In the realm of wealth and finance, this is the quadrant where Mr. Pretender realizes that his financial situation is not what he thought it was. He makes a determination to be like Mr. Rich. He moves into a smaller house and trades in his expensive cars for more economical ones (these are like using medications and surgeries in health) to reduce the expenses. But he doesn't stop there. He also creates "wealth assets."

For example, with the extra money left from the sale of his big house, he buys a small rental property to bring in extra income. By doing both, his progress will be faster toward becoming like Mr. Rich. If he fails to create positive cash flow, and only depends on economizing, his progress will be slow, and another economic collapse can result in another major setback.

It is the same in health. If we do not engage in activities to rebalance the generation-to-depletion ratio, any other adverse force can easily make itself at home in our body. This is why, during the pandemic, the government and fake health system announced that people with underlying medical conditions are at high risk of dying from COVID-19. Yet, I have seen some people with underlying conditions survive the virus, and others who did not. Although both groups of people were in the same "E" quadrant, they were at different levels of balance within that quadrant (Figure 10.3). This is similar to the differential balance of those that had complete recovery or developed post COVID-19 syndrome discussed under "I" quadrant.

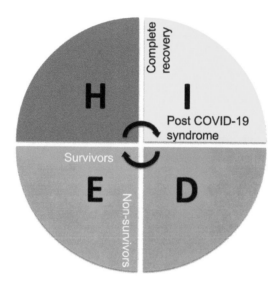

Figure 10.3: Position of the differential balance in "I" and "E" quadrants.

The disparity depended on the ratio they had established while remaining in this quadrant. For example, people whose vital-force generation far exceeded depletion had enough reserve to overcome the additional infection while those who barely generated what they depleted succumb to it. It's almost like those that survived were rapidly moving within "E" quadrant closer to "H" quadrant while those that did not survive remained closer to "D" quadrant with regard to the generation-to-depletion ratio (Figure 10.3). Both were in the same "E" quadrant, albeit with different generation-to-depletion ratio. If you find yourself in this quadrant, whether you are closer to "H" or "D" depends on your daily effort.

CHAPTER 11

Cognizance: Can everyone become aware of the true self?

Awareness

Having dealt with the misdirected focus of health for so long, change requires reprograming our silent partner to a correct idea of health. Awareness is embedded in the recognition for change. Self-awareness is at the center of success or failure in any aspect of life, and is the same in relation to success and failure in health. We have the power to change what we're aware of, whereas anything we are not aware of has the power to change us. Most often, we're not even aware of the inner battles we are fighting every day.

> *We define what we are aware of,*
> *and what we are unaware defines us.*

Chapter 10 dealt with the transition of our health status in response to the balance between positive and negative life-flow. Awareness of the transition from the "H" quadrant to the "I" quadrant makes us more successful, because it promotes us to take action to prevent moving in the wrong direction. If, by chance, we contracted a disease, awareness is required to move from the "D" to the "E" quadrant. Most often, when we speak of health, our focus is entirely on one area—our physical bodies.

Let's be honest: up until this point, while reading this book, your internal awareness may be reflexively relating this information to your physical body. It's only natural; after all, that's how we've trained ourselves. Our physical body is the most tangible aspect of our self, and that which is the most tangible is the easiest to comprehend. For that reason, it's imperative that, as Abraham Maslow said, we become fully aware of all that constitutes us—the human self.

Fake Self

We are complex beings. Trying to make sense out of all the layers that we call our self and the interactions of those layers within us and outside of us is a monumental task. At age seventeen, I was presented with the most complicated question of my life, asked of me by a guru as I was being initiated into yoga and meditation: "Who are you?"

I was dumbfounded, as the guru already knew who I was. Thinking it was a ritual, I mentioned my name and my family line and a few characteristics that defined me. The guru smiled at me and said, "That is a good start, but is incorrect." He said, "That is your identity, your fake self, not who you are. Look beyond your identity, beyond your fake self. Look within. Keep asking yourself this question as you go through the practice of meditation and the answer will reveal itself."

Ever since that day, I embarked on an exploration of "who I am" by observing myself in addition to others, especially patients who were close to death. Patients close to death begin to lose their worldly identity and begin to manifest their true being. At this point a person's silent partner has no real purpose or value. Because silent partner is about how we live. I read scientific literature on personality and human behavior, and went on to learn Buddhism and Christianity in search of an answer. The answer has yet to be fully revealed to me after twenty-five years of study, reflection, and self-observation. But my efforts did enable self-growth and recognition of something else when I had a brush with death during my heart attack.

The idea of my personal identity and everything I believed I knew about me was rendered useless at that time. I needed to let go of the existing reality and surrender to a deeper presence within myself. It was that surrender—not my knowledge as a cardiologist, not the technological wonder of modern medicine, not my fake identity—that came to the rescue.

After that brush with death, one thing became clear: there is a presence, a being, within us, that reveals itself when worldly pretentions about us disappear. Pretentions about us usually disappear at extreme desperate situations. That deeper presence is not the same as what we call our self, "I." "I" refers to the superficial and pretentious manifestations that we consciously believe to be our own selves and project to the world. In essence there are three layers of self; an inner self, an outer self, and a fake self. These three layers consist of their own layers as depicted in Figures 11.1 & 11.2.

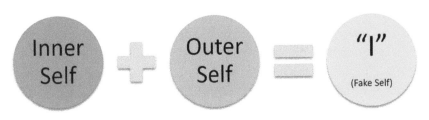

Figure 11.1: The three layers of our total self.

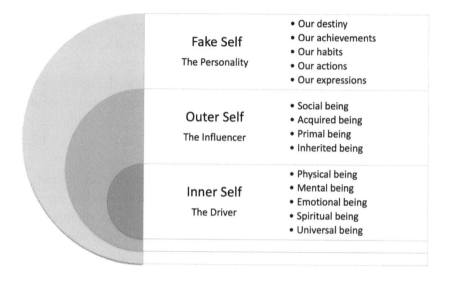

Fake Self The Personality	• Our destiny • Our achievements • Our habits • Our actions • Our expressions
Outer Self The Influencer	• Social being • Acquired being • Primal being • Inherited being
Inner Self The Driver	• Physical being • Mental being • Emotional being • Spiritual being • Universal being

Figure 11.2: The three selves and their individual components.

I had to let go of the fake self and outer self in order to reach the deeper presence. This deeper presence functions below our conscious level, and gives origin to deeper drives. Those deeper drives are modified at conscious level through several layers prior to being expressed as part of our fake self in the outer world (Figure 11.4). Logical brain and silent partner strongly modify these deeper drives and convert them into our superficial outer world manifestations—the "I," our personality, the fake self. From there, we continue our interaction primarily with our silent partner, who is a component of our outer self. We don't look beyond silent partner into the drive that gave rise to that outer world manifestation. In daily life, therefore, the immediate engagement with our silent partner prevents us from looking beyond the superficial manifestations to the deeper presence within.

As a result, we live with multiple identities created by our silent partner, and miss the true self, that deeper presence, the spirit. The spontaneous and immediate engagement of the silent partner, at the time the drive of an inner being hits our awareness, masks the origin of that inner drive and alters our recognition of that drive. If we train our awareness to prevent the immediate engagement of the silent partner, we are a step closer to the true self.

In fact, there are nine identifiable beings that influence our personality (Figure 11.3). We recognize the collective product of these beings as the self, which we call "I" or "ME." *This "I" or "ME" is a fake identification of who we are.* This was the identification I gave the guru when he asked who I was, and it was the identification that dissolved at the time of my heart attack. All those years in between, I continued to misidentify the derivative—personality—as the true being. The "I," our personality and the fake self are one and the same.

There are five inner beings that make up our inner self, and four outer beings that make up our outer self. The interactions of these beings with our deeper drives generate our personality—our fake self—for the outer world. Our true self, that inner presence, is hidden deep within our universal being. I had to let go of even my physical, mental, emotional, and spiritual levels of the inner self and transcend to the universal level to connect with my deeper presence—spirit.

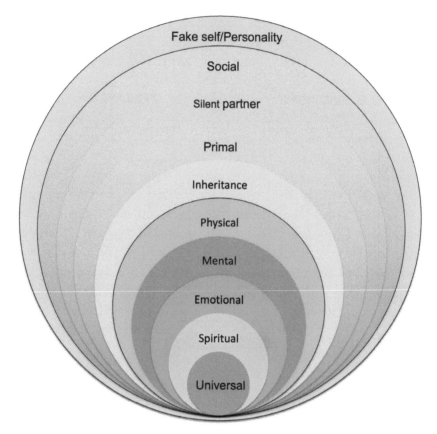

Figure 11.3: The layers of human unit.

It's easy to let go of the physical, mental, emotional, and spiritual levels when death seems imminent. It's harder on a day-to-day basis when faced with life's distractions. Our true self lies deeper than the fake self and the outer self; it lies at the depth of our inner self. One has to let go of the personality and the beings that generate that personality to reveal the true self.

Battle of the Beings

We not only interact with the outer world, but also interact with the world within ourselves. We are mostly aware of our interaction of the fake self with the outer world, and are ignorant to the interactions that go on within our outer and inner selves. The five beings or intelligences of the inner self are projections of our spirit (we previously discussed the phenomenon of the transfer of these intelligences between humans via organ transplant in Chapter 8).

The drives of these five inner beings is filtered through the four outer beings—our outer self—manifesting as our personality (our fake self) in the outer world (Figure 11.4). This is important because in order to change our personality/behavior, we have to be aware of the drivers and influencers behind that behavior.

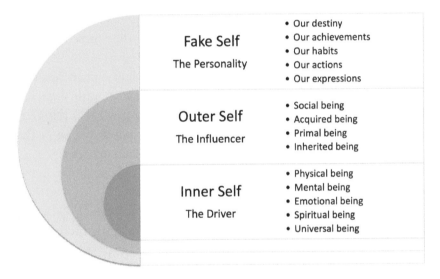

Figure11.4: Deep drives and impulses of inner self ascend and are filtered through several layers.

In the course of our lives, we collectively consider our body and mind as one, and refer to it as I or ME and not as being comprised of several layers. When an impulse arising at our inner self finally arrives at conscious level as a thought, our silent partner is immediately engaged. Silent partner further modifies and influences that original thought prior to us making a decision on an action based on that thought. If we can train ourselves to figure out the level of origin of the impulse prior to allowing silent partner to engage, clarity in thinking can be achieved. Clear thinking leads to clearly defined actions. Clearly defined actions enhance the chance of success.

Health abilities are developed through behavior. It is, therefore, important to understand the beings that influence our behavior in order to master health. While I still don't know the answer to the question "Who are you?" I believe that I do know where the barriers are that prevent us from connecting with the real self. It is within us. The key to our success or failure lies in the layers that constitute our body-mind interaction as depicted in Figure 11.3. The layers that lie within us interact with each other not in a linear fashion but simultaneously in a complex fashion. Years of exploration into the true self has led to a simplified comprehension of how the inner and outer selves interact with each other, and in turn how they present within us and to the outside world.

This understanding is portrayed in the body-mind interaction triangle (BMIT) illustrated below. The human unit depicted in Figure 11.3 is like anatomy of our total self and what is depicted in BMIT is like the functional arrangement of our self. Use of the BMIT greatly enhances our understanding of human behavior. In addition to facilitating the understanding of ourselves, it also facilitates the understanding of people we interact with.

In *Second Opinion*, the same triangle is named the HI (Human Interaction) triangle. In this book, the triangle is slightly modified to illustrate the role of the acquired being—our silent partner and the resulting social being. A full discussion on the nine beings and their interaction within us is beyond the scope of this book, however, a brief description of the levels of being is addressed below.

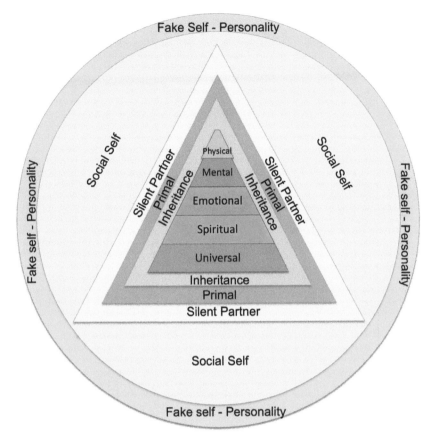

Figure 11.5: The Body-Mind Interaction Triangle (BMIT) illustrating the interaction of the beings.

The Inner Self

The Physical Being

Definition: Having material existence; perceptible especially through the senses and subject to the laws of nature or relating to the body.

The physical being relates to our body and its functions. This level communicates with us through our five senses. Symptoms such as aches and pains, nausea, shortness of breath, etc., are all part of the physical level. This is the most tangible of all levels of our inner self.

Most often, when we think of health, our awareness focuses on this level of being only. Medicine directs its focus on disease and its symptoms, which confines our attention to this level only. That is one of the reasons why we cannot successfully achieve and maintain health with modern medicine.

People who are athletically inclined predominantly excel at and manifest this level—their physical being. That doesn't mean they don't function on other levels, only that they tend to nurture and manifest their physical being in particular. The physical being is their direct visible truth because that level dominates their awareness. *The complex interaction of all aspects that relate to our physical sensations is termed physical intelligence.* (Further reading: *Sensation: The New Science of Physical Intelligence* by Prof. Thalma Lobel.) Physical intelligence operates our physical being.

The Mental Being

Definition: Of or relating to intellectual as contrasted with emotional or physical activity.

This level represents our feelings and thoughts (intellectual activity). We may or may not be consciously aware of each and every one of these thoughts. When we study a subject or have intellectual discussions, we are involving our mental being in that activity.

Physicians, lawyers, accountants, engineers, philosophers, and professors are all examples of people who predominantly exercise their mental being; their activities are mainly intellectual in nature. Again, just because they predominantly function from this level does not mean they do not exhibit other levels of being. It just means that they predominantly nurture and manifest their mental being. *The complex interaction of all aspects that relates to intellectual activity is termed mental intelligence.* Mental intelligence operates our mental being.

The Emotional Being

Definition: A conscious mental reaction (such as anger or fear) subjectively experienced as strong feeling usually directed toward a specific object and typically accompanied by physiological and behavioral changes in the body.

Emotions are reactions to an internal or external stimulus, and occur fleetingly (because it is a reaction). For example, fear of falling ill from COVID-19 drove people to social distance. Emotion is "energy in motion." This is because, when the internal or external stimulus triggers an emotion, it is accompanied by a biological reaction and sets the internal environment (our terrain) in motion. This biological reaction is usually a predecessor to an action. For example, in a fight or flight situation, fear (emotion) causes the heart rate and blood pressure to rise and the palms to sweat (biological reaction) in preparation for fight or flight (action).

Emotions frequently dictate our actions by engaging our silent partner, irrespective of whether they are positive or negative. When someone's long-term actions are driven from the emotional plane, they begin to identify themselves with this plane. That becomes their direct and visible truth. The other planes become less visible as the emotional plane continues to drive them. For example, artists, singers, and actors are some examples of professionals that predominantly function from and manifest this level of our being. *The body of complex interactions that leads to this manifestation is called emotional intelligence.*

The Spiritual Being

Definition: The inner character of a person; thought of as different from the material person we can see and touch.

The above definition implies that this plane is related to the spirit of human beings (the vital-force). The spirit resides in the universal level. The spiritual being is the unadulterated manifestation of that spirit. It is important to understand that the existence and manifestation of spirit in us is at two different levels. The spiritual being can be influenced by the religion of a person (Figure 11.6), but this level exists in all of us, irrespective of what religion we belong to (or don't belong to).

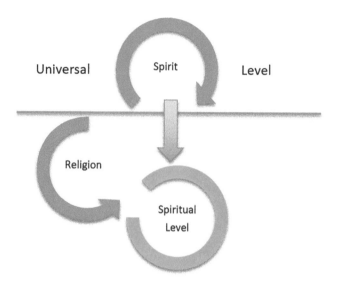

Figure 11.6: Relationship between human spirit at universal level, religion, and spiritual level.

This level is devoid of sensations, thoughts, or emotions. In the BMIT, it is placed just above the level of "unknown," and just below the other three levels. It acts as the doorway to the "unknown" level. This is the level where we may feel a "notion," but we cannot describe it in words. This is the level of intuition—the ability to immediately understand something without conscious reasoning.

Without being able to describe an intuition, the mental level cannot process it. As a result, we cannot act on it other than just waiting for that "intuition" to manifest. When an act is performed from this level, nothing is expected in return because there is no logical understanding of that act. This level is selfless, unlike the physical, mental, or emotional planes, which are processed at conscious level and are selfish. The manifestation of spiritual being results in selfless giving. A good example of a person who embodied and manifested this level of being is Mother Teresa.

Have you ever heard someone say, "Follow your heart" or "I am making the decision with my heart and not my head"? When someone refers to their "head," they're referring to the physical, emotional, or mental level—conscious reasoning. When we follow our head, we can logically explain our decision. On the other hand, when we follow our "heart," we only have a sense of what direction we want to go.

Put simply, if we follow our head, we have the roadmap before the journey starts. If we follow the heart, we draw the roadmap as we go along. Consequently, following the heart (functioning from the spiritual being) requires tremendous courage arising from faith.

Oftentimes, when we think we're following the heart, it leads to a disastrous outcome. This is because we've misidentified the drives from the emotional plane as coming from the spiritual plane. This mistake is frequently made because we mistakenly associate the heart with emotions. If we truly followed the heart, as it's meant to be followed, we will be successful in whatever we do.

When we function mainly from the spiritual plane, we identify ourselves as spiritual beings, because that is the direct and visible truth. The other planes are less manifested in our consciousness. Religion has a powerful influence on this plane.

For centuries, wars have been fought in the name of religion. Through wars and civil unrest, we are still experiencing the misdirected power of this plane across the globe.

Religious leaders, pastors, priests, yogis, charity workers, true philanthropists, and volunteer workers are all examples of people mainly exercising the spiritual level. *The complex mechanism of interaction that leads from the awareness of that "sense" to the action is the spiritual intelligence.*

The Universal Being

Definition: Lacking material substance; of or relating to the regions beyond the earth. Seeming to belong to another world, e.g.: heaven. This being is also referred to as the "unknown being" in this book.

Every day, we interact with this level without being aware of it. This plane pertains to the uncertainty beyond our control. For example, there are people who pray before going to bed that they will wake up the next morning. How certain are we that we will wake up the next morning? The answer is, "Not certain."

We do not stop to question the momentary awareness of this being when it flashes across our mind. Whenever our mind responds with, "I don't know," we are dealing with the unknown level. It applies to everything that involves chance in life. Even in health, chance plays a major role. Chance played a role in who contracted COVID-19, and who lived or died. Social distancing was about reducing the chance of contracting the virus, but it was still a matter of chance. The whole system of biostatistics was developed to address this unknown level. Yet, we ignore this level in our daily life.

If you are someone who reads daily horoscopes, you are consciously seeking to address this unknown. If you go to the psychic for predictions of the future, you are consciously trying to reveal this level. If you are consulting with a lawyer or your accountant to find out "the risk" before embarking on a new business venture or pursuit, you are dealing with this level. If you ask your doctor how successful the medication or the proposed surgery is going to be, you are dealing with this level. Our daily life is filled with it. This being is the driver of all of those above actions, yet, how many of us fully recognize it?

Some people call it the "universal consciousness," "universal energy," "universal power," "ethereal level," or "God." No matter what name is used, it is there in our life and is part of our functioning, despite whether we choose to acknowledge it or not. In my opinion, it's the most powerful of all the planes discussed in this chapter. It's important to note that this plane is part of us, but it does not exclusively belong to us: it is universal. All human beings share this plane.

Faith is the tool that connects us to this level. The word faith appeals to us irrespective of color, creed, or nationality. It appeals to the deepest player of all: the spirit. The reason that religions are so prevalent and powerful is because they connect us to the unknown through faith. All religions are about faith.

Deep down, we feel the drive of this level at all times, but it's not brought into full awareness because it's not formulated into thoughts and words. Instead, the universal level manifests through others, and once it's animated, it animates the other eight beings also. The continuous chatter of the other beings masks the message from the universal level, preventing it from reaching our awareness.

However, with practice, such as through meditation, we can learn to interact with this level if we choose to.

The universal level provides power and intensity for our intentions. When an emotion is strong enough to result in an intention, the continued power to maintain that intention is derived from this level. Therefore, this universal level plays a key role in our accomplishments, irrespective of whether the accomplishment is intended to be positive or negative. The alignment of our intention with our silent partner and spirit (emanating from this level) is a powerful combination.

We discussed this power in Chapter 7. When the spirit and intentions align, we appear to have the power to accomplish whatever we want. When someone accomplishes a seemingly impossible feat, it then becomes more easily achievable by those that follow.

The example of Roger Bannister, the twenty-five-year-old medical student who broke the four-minute mile, is one such example. The expressions, "If there's a will there's a way," and, "Be careful what you wish for," are related to this level.

People who primarily function from the other levels still have the ability to tap into this unknown level. Successful athletes (physical plane), entrepreneurs (mental plane), artists (emotional plane), and enlightened spiritual leaders (spiritual plane) are all examples of people who function primarily from other planes, but all have found success by tapping into the power of the unknown level.

This is why engaging the spirit is an important aspect of health. I call functioning from this level *"functioning in the grey zone,"* because the drive is not black and white to our conscious mind as it is based on faith. *The complex mechanism that animates this level is the universal intelligence.*

The Outer Self

Most of our drives that arise from any level of the BMIT are influenced by all four of the gatekeepers depicted in the triangle: primal, acquired (silent partner), social, and inherited. These gatekeepers modify how the drives of the five inner beings are expressed under the guidance of the silent partner and how they present to the world.

The Inherited Being

When we speak of genetics, we're referring to the physical and psychological traits we inherited from our parents. We are predisposed to be healthy, unhealthy, or prone to developing diseases based on what we inherit. The natural tendency of our body is to be healthy and in balance. Just because we have a predisposition for a particular disease, does not mean we have to develop that disease in our lifetime. I have seen some patients who do, and others who do not. *This inheritance influences "who we are," but it does not dictate who we should be.*

For example, it has been shown that middle-aged men who perform moderate exercise on a regular basis (such as thirty minutes of brisk walking six days a week) tend to have a longer life. This is because of the effect that exercise has on an area of our chromosomes called the "telomere." Telomeres are the protective end-caps of chromosomes that determine how quickly our cells age. These telomeres are composed of DNA and proteins, and they protect and stabilize the ends of the chromosome from degrading. Telomeres shorten over time, so longer telomeres equate to longer cell-life. But lifestyle changes in men with prostate cancer have been shown to increase (ten percent increase over five years) the length of the telomeres, conferring a better prognosis compared to groups that didn't make the lifestyle changes (this group had a three percent reduction in the length of their telomere over a five-year period) (Ornish, 2008).

In addition, emotions have been shown to influence genetics in such a way that even without genetic predisposition, disease manifested after being subjected to certain emotional stressors. (Recommended reading: *Change Your Genes Change Your Life* by Dr. Kenneth Pelletier.) In other words, our genetics are in constant interaction with the five levels of being. Therefore, modification of our five inner beings can modify our inherited traits.

The Primal Being

Primal, in this context, means "basic" or "primary," and refers to our unfiltered and unmodified being. This being consists of the unfiltered drives related to our basic existence and desires. These include: hunger, sex, elimination, sleep, survival (aggression), and socialization. A child exhibits these drives in the most primitive fashion. A child will cry for food when hungry; they have no inhibition.

When we grow up, we still carry those primal drives, but we don't manifest them to society in an unfiltered fashion. We modify those drives (this modified version is the subject of the next section, "social being"). In adults, the primal being refers to our wants, thoughts, and actions when we're in private, as opposed to what we express and manifest in the presence of others. If we are in a social setting, our primal being is still present internally, despite what we present to those around us.

What I've described as the primal being closely resembles what Sigmund Freud described as the "Id." However, the primal being not only includes the instinctual drives attributed to the "Id," but also the unfiltered drives toward doing anything.

These additional drives include the desire to become rich, an entrepreneur, an Olympian, a leader in your company, a boss, etc.

I believe that our drives for action come from the five levels that have been previously described. If one's primal being is stronger than the social being, most of one's actions would be reflected outwardly without much filter and modification.

The Social Being

The social being is the filtered, or modified, side of us, the side that we project to the world irrespective of what we're inwardly thinking. This is the being that we spend a considerable amount of time trying to perfect. All of our drives, including the primal being, are ultimately expressed to society through the social being. The way we dress, the way we speak, how we observe etiquettes, and how we adjust our mannerisms in different situations are all examples of the manifestation of our social being.

The social being is the manifestation that Sigmund Freud described as the "ego." It is the filtered part of our personality, modified to be acceptable to society. Potty training is an example of taming the primal being, so that it can be presented in a socially acceptable way. The social being never replaces the primal being. Rather, the primal being slowly learns to manifest as a social being through reinforcement by society.

The Acquired Being – Silent Partner

Our silent partner is like a computer algorithm programmed to influence the unfiltered drive for action. The silent partner, as mentioned before, consists of our cultural, religious, and ethnic values that we have learned from parents, teachers, religious leaders, peers, and role models. These values are internalized, and heavily influence how our drives are expressed through actions.

The silent partner is our value system, or "internal compass." I call this "our rules of engagement" and they pertain to every aspect of our life. The silent partner makes up the majority of our conscience. It's the part of our psyche that differentiates right or wrong and punishes misbehavior. Some confuse the silent partner with conscience. Unadulterated conscience already exists when we are born. We modify the conscience with acquired training as we grow and this acquired body of information that shapes how our conscience functions are what I call silent partner. The silent partner is the genesis of our opinions. For example, while reading this book, if we are thinking that the material contained in the book is bull, it is an opinion, while our conscience may actually be aligned with what we are reading. Our silent partner just gave us an opinion. Silent partner is embedded in our conscience. We deepen the duality of conscience through our acquired body of information called silent partner. Therefore, our opinions and decisions depend on what kind of information has been acquired by the silent partner, which in turn depends on how we grew up.

The words *Id*, *Ego*, and *Super-ego* translate in English into the following:

- Id = the "It"
- Ego = the "I"
- Super-ego = The "over I" or the "above I"

These original words are pretty self-explanatory. As a result, one can perceive the super-ego as the supervisor (above "I") of the other two (the "It" and the "I"). The supervisor influences the manifestation of the other two; therefore, the supervisor is not visible to the outside world. The super-ego is responsible for justifying our ideas of right and wrong, and is responsible for our social appropriateness. While the id demands unfiltered desire for instant gratification, the super-ego strives for perfection and socially acceptable behavior. They therefore tend to contradict each other.

The ego acts as the mediator between the two; it seeks to satisfy the demands of both the id and the super-ego. The better developed our ego, the better refined we are in expressing our primal drives to the outer world. The ego may have difficulty reconciling the demands of the id and super-ego—this is the beginning of a conflict in a person.

I believe that the conflict of the ego is a very important concept in health and disease. In my opinion, a conflict is the very first step in which an imbalance begins. With time, this imbalance drains life-flow and reduces vital-force, predisposing us to disease. The individual who later develops the disease may not even remember the start of the conflict; this is why we don't recognize the conflict as the instigator for the disease.

Modern medicine falls far behind in identifying this point in the disease process. On the other hand, traditional, alternative, and complementary medicine are all about identifying this imbalance.

The Balance of the Terrain

Health is the ability to maintain and re-establish the balance of the internal environment. The components of our internal environment, or "terrain" as described by Claude Bernard, was not detailed in previous chapters. The purpose of this chapter was to illustrate the components that constitute our internal environment. Humans can establish and maintain the balance of the different beings of the inner self (drives) by modifying the outer self (influencer), leading to a change in behavior (personality).

Successful people are able to accomplish this task by predominantly retraining their acquired being/silent partner for long-lasting results. Additionally, achieving and maintaining balance of each level, as well as balance between levels, is essential to continue creating vital-force and life-flow, leading to a formidable health reserve.

CHAPTER 12

Continuation: Can everyone renew health?

Hidden in Plain Sight

Human beings are, by nature, energetic beings. Whether the spirit is manifesting our physical, mental, emotional, or spiritual being at any given moment depends on which being is contacted and energized. Our body manifests as matter to the naked eye, but hidden within that matter is a profound power that is largely unrecognized. This energy expresses itself through one of our five beings. Science tells us that anything that transforms is energetic in nature. As human beings, we are constantly transforming, in ways largely unbeknownst to us. It is important to recognize that even something that we are unaware of has the power to change our destiny.

Spontaneous Health Renewal

The idea that health is renewable by choice sounds preposterous. But if we think in terms of the currency of health—vital-force—and the regeneration of vital- force, the idea is more palatable. Our cells consume energy to live, and generate more to keep us alive. Considered macroscopically, the human body consumes energy (food) to sustain life, and in turn, generates the energy needed to perform the daily tasks of living. The function of the human body is the result of the collective function of the cells that make up the body. We have to choose actions that promote vital-force renewal in our cells and minimize actions that deplete vital-force or prevent our cells from generating it.

Not everyone is aware of the ability to renew health, though some discover it through their own observation. I've met patients who recognized this potential after heart transplant, and some who recognized it before transplant (and were then able to avoid transplant altogether). My personal recognition comes from observing thousands of patients, myself included, as well as through my education in both Eastern and Western concepts of health and disease. Others recognized it in the brush with a life-threatening disease. But not everyone has to go through these processes. An active decision and subsequent commitment is all that's needed.

We renew health every single day without being aware of the fact it is health that we are renewing. When we've depleted our energy at the end of the day and go to sleep, we wake up with recovered energy the next morning. Sleeping, eating, breathing, and our heartbeat all help renew our energy. Most of these actions are taken for granted.

When the heart cannot effectively pump, it cannot effectively assist the renewal of energy, and life is shortened. It's the same with our lungs. When lung disease develops, we cannot effectively renew energy via oxygen exchange, and our life is shortened. The kidneys and liver work tirelessly to help remove toxins that reduce generation of energy. Our gut does both, separating food from toxins, using the fuel for energy and eliminating the toxins from our body. We even have bacteria in our guts—"cohabitants" that help us renew health.

The renewal described above is *spontaneous health renewal by our body*, and the body performs these functions without extra effort from us. While we can't re-program these functions, we can influence them for short periods at a time. This can be done through actions such as holding our breath, intermittent fasting, elevating our heart rate, bowel cleansing, and pulling all-nighters. If we over- or under-perform these activities, it becomes an adverse force because it violates the laws of nature. For example, inadequate or excessive fasting, eating, exercising, breathing, colonic cleansing, and sleeping are detrimental to our health because they upset the very balance we are trying to maintain. Nature seeks balance.

Cultivated Health Renewal

As opposed to spontaneous renewal, there is also *cultivated health renewal,* which can be actively accomplished. For example, physical rehabilitation is prescribed after a surgery or prolonged illness to renew the patient's health. This is achieved by recovering the energy that was spent by the illness. Through rehabilitation, health is renewed to a point where a person can create a new balance—a new normal.

This renewability is what helps people move from the Disease ("D") quadrant to the Equilibrium ("E") quadrant. Mr. Lazy had to go through rehabilitative renewal to become eligible for heart transplant. He didn't completely recover from his heart condition, but by improving his health reserve through rehabilitation, he became strong enough to undergo heart transplant surgery. He increased his internal environment's vital-force enough to ensure that the transplanted heart could successfully embed and survive.

Duality

Anything that is in balance has duality—up and down. The word "balance" or "equilibrium" is the key. Health is maintained moment-to-moment and is experienced moment-to-moment in everything we do. For example, how do we perceive we have a disease or an illness? Because disease makes us aware of itself by producing symptoms such as aches and pains, tiredness, upset belly, etc. These symptoms can be present during every moment of our wakeful state. Isn't that why we seek help to alleviate those symptoms, so that we can feel comfortable? We feel disease because the symptoms of disease constantly nag us unless we take medications to mask them.

Likewise, health is also a constant experience, though we don't pay attention to what it feels like until we lose it. We accept it as our normal state and take it for granted. Unfortunately, most of us don't pay attention when we lose health, either. This is because we've been trained by fake health to recognize the rise of disease, but not the loss of health. Hence our dependency on medications, surgeries, and quick-fix methods—forgetting the best tool we have: ourselves.

Eastern traditions like Ayurveda recognized the existence of vital-force, and called it "prana." In the West, the concept of spirit remains abstract, and is ignored by modern medicine. It was Chinese medicine that refined the idea of vital-force as having duality. Ancient Chinese thinking recognized duality in nature—the opposing and complementary characteristics in everything they observed in the world around us. Based on this, they named certain characteristics of nature as "Yang," and the opposite characteristics as "Yin." The concept of duality implies three phenomena.

First: there are always two sides to anything (feelings, emotions, organic and inorganic matters, etc.). It's almost like "the opposites game" played in pre-school.

Second: the natural state is for these two sides to be in equilibrium—they are well-balanced in their opposition to one another.

Third: due to the tendency to be in equilibrium, these two aspects are complementary to each other. One cannot exist without the other—there cannot be night without the existence of day.

It's similar to the two sides of a coin. If we are looking at one side of the coin, we inherently know there is another side, even though we aren't focusing on the other side at that particular moment. A coin cannot exist without having both sides, and it's perfectly balanced when the two sides are equal in every aspect. One side of the coin is "Yin" and the other is "Yang." All matter, living or not, has this complementary duality called Yin and Yang. A few examples of Yin and Yang are given in the table below.

Phenomenon	Yin	Yang
Celestial bodies	Moon	Sun
Time of day	Night	Day
Gender	Female	Male
Location	Inside	Outside
Temperature	Cold	Hot
Direction	Downward	Upward
Degree of humidity	Damp/Moist	Dry
Color	Black	White

Table 12.1: The concept of Yin and Yang.

Nature constantly exhibits this balance of opposing and complementary features. Approximately seventy percent of the Earth's surface is water, and coincidentally, so is seventy percent of the human body. The molecules of water do not sit still. Our health is the same: the vital-force does not sit still. Water can assume three states. It can be a liquid, solid, or a vapor.

In Table 12.1, hot is designated *Yang*, and cold is designated *Yin*. Steam is the most Yang state of water, and ice is its most Yin state. In its most Yin state (ice), the water is inert and less energized. In its most Yang state (steam), it is dynamic and more energized. While steam and ice have their purposes in nature, a state of fluidity (liquid) is the most versatile and useful form. When fluid, water's Yang and Yin aspects are in equilibrium.

Even in its fluid state, water can exhibit its Yin and Yang characteristics and still be in equilibrium. Take ocean water for example. The surface of the ocean has dynamic waves, but deep below the surface, the water is still. In both of these areas, the ocean is fluid, yet, it exhibits its Yang (waves) and its Yin (stillness) characteristics simultaneously. We can see that the water has duality (Yin and Yang) while remaining in its perfectly balanced fluid state.

Our bodies are naturally designed to be in just such a perfectly balanced state. If the water's equilibrium is lost and the Yang aspect prevails, water loses its calmness and becomes rough and turbulent. If it becomes more Yin, it freezes and becomes icy. In mental health, it's like having bipolar disorder. In its extreme Yang, the disorder is in its manic phase, and in its extreme Yin, it exhibits major depression.

The calm and navigable ocean (the balanced state where the Yin and Yang are in equilibrium) is most useful for sailors. Rough water and ice are dangerous and not conducive to smooth sailing. Obviously, we cannot control the external Yin/Yang of water, but in health, we do have control of our internal Yin/Yang—just as a sailor cannot control the water, but they can control the sail of the boat to navigate the water.

The sailor seeks advice from the coast guard when they're unsure of the water's conditions, and similarly, we seek help from a medical practitioner when we are feeling "off" or are exhibiting symptoms of disease. In life, the question for us is whether we want to control the water or the sail. Most of us try to control the water and that's why we fail. Success is achieved by learning how to control the sail.

During the 2020 pandemic, those that were in a balanced state were healthy and sailed smoothly—they had control of their own sail. During the same period, those that were in an unbalanced state were unhealthy and had rough sailing—they relied on controlling external factors beyond their control.

The Two Aspects of the Vital-Force

The behavior of vital-force in humans is no different than the water example above. Vital-force has two attributes: one that is dynamic/renewable (Yang), and one that is static/non-renewable (Yin). The dynamic attribute engages with any activity related to the survival of the organism, while the static attribute does not, but serves as a reserve (Figure 12.1 below). These two components are part of the same vital-force, but they exhibit two different characteristics—Yin (non-renewable) and Yang (renewable). Applying this to the ocean example, the dynamic waves are like the renewable portion of the vital-force, and the static depth is like the non-renewable portion of the vital-force. Yet, these two portions belong to the same ocean.

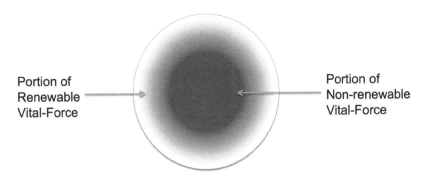

Figure 12.1: The concept of renewable and non-renewable portions of the same vital-force.

The renewable component of vital-force is constantly engaged in animating the activities of our total being that includes maintaining a healthy state. Sustaining life is dynamic by definition because of its active engagement. Any part of the vital-force can switch between renewable and non-renewable at any moment (white arrows in Figure 12.2 below), just as the water from the ocean's depth (Yin) can move to the surface and become a wave (Yang) and vice-versa.

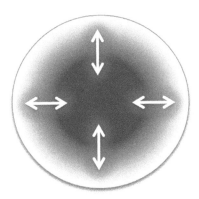

Figure 12.2: Constant exchange of vital-force between renewable and non-renewable portions.

Yin and Yang are characteristics, or attributes, of all aspects in life. In both vital-force, as in water, the attributes are either dynamic or sluggish, and the medium continuously changes its attributes to maintain balance.

With regard to vital-force, the issue to consider is that the dynamically engaged (renewable/Yang) attribute yields itself to change through our behavior (just like the surface Yang of the ocean yields to a sailor's ability to navigate their ship). When an ocean's Yin or Yang is off-balance and the ocean becomes turbulent, the sailor will have difficulties navigating. Likewise, if our vital-force's Yin or Yang is off-balance (disequilibrium), we will not function properly.

When we feel "a little off" with mild aches and pains, slight sluggishness, minor headaches, lack of appetite, or difficulty sleeping, it means that our equilibrium of vital-force is off. If these feelings persist, we move from the Healthy ("H") quadrant to the Imbalance ("I") quadrant. If we allow ourselves to continue in this quadrant, we develop disease and move from the Imbalance ("I") quadrant to the Disease ("D") quadrant.

The good news is we can deliberately influence the equilibrium, but first we need to learn how to navigate this renewable vital-force.

Adverse forces negatively affect this renewable portion and deplete our energy—resulting in negative life-flow. In finance, these adverse forces are called liabilities (causing negative cash flow), and in health, they're called *health liabilities*. On the other hand, actions that positively affect and increase vital-force are *health assets* and lead to positive life-flow (positive cash flow with regard to wealth).

Health assets increase the renewable energy and thereby promote stronger equilibrium between the Yin and Yang aspect of the vital-force. *Stated simply, any action or event that puts more energy into us is a health asset and any action that takes energy out of us is a health liability.* The stronger the equilibrium of the vital-force, the stronger the equilibrium of the person, and as a result, the stronger the health reserve. The reverse is true when the vital-force energy is in disequilibrium.

The water example above clarifies the dual nature of our vital-force. The portion of energy that engages and supports our activities is dynamic and therefore Yang. This dynamic portion is the renewable aspect of the vital-force. When we're engaged with health liabilities, we constantly lose energy from this dynamic portion. In order to be balanced, this loss needs to be minimized, and whatever was lost needs to be replaced. The concept of continuous renewal and positive life-flow by health assets and negative life-flow by health liabilities is illustrated below (Figure 12.3).

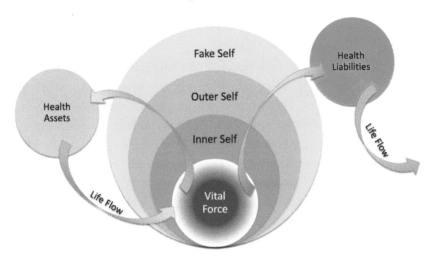

Figure 12.3: Pattern of life-flow renewal and depletion as it relates to health assets, liabilities and the three selves.

Let us consider another example. Consider a piece of land in our backyard where we want to grow a garden. The entire backyard is vast, so we allocate a small portion of it for cultivating. We prepare the land and plant whatever we like. The garden needs constant attention: watering, weeding, weather protection, pest control, etc. If our attention fails, the garden will lose its optimal capacity to grow, but if we dedicate the utmost attention and care, we reap maximum benefit.

The garden is like the renewable dynamic portion of vital-force. The rest of the backyard also belongs to us, but is not actively cultivated, and is like the non-renewable portion of vital-force.

Even though the entire backyard is not actively cultivated, it could be cultivated at any time. For example, if we deplete all the nutrients from the current garden, we can pick another piece of the backyard for gardening. The garden is like our own health: it is renewed as long as we keep maintaining it.

If we do not maintain it, the garden declines over time, just like our health. At this point, we have to tap into the rest of the land and start cultivating there to regain those benefits. Having to tap into the new portion of land is like having to establish a new balance when we develop disease. It is like moving from the Disease ("D") quadrant to the Equilibrium ("E") quadrant.

When we pick a new portion of the backyard to cultivate, it becomes the dynamic Yang aspect—the renewable portion. Without careful maintenance, this process can go on and on until all of the land is depleted of nutrients and becomes useless. If this happens with our vital-force, we move into the Disease ("D") quadrant with an end-stage disease like heart, kidney, liver failure, or cancer. At this point, trying to maintain the garden is not enough. We may need pesticides (similar to using modern medicine against disease), and then continue to strengthen the land with nutrient-rich fertilizer (similar to health assets) to prevent further infestation.

Patients who receive a heart transplant are given a second chance at life from the new, donated heart. This is like being given a new piece of land to cultivate. After heart transplant, I have seen some patients realize their mistakes, and convert to using more health assets to care for their new inheritance. I've also seen patients who continue to indulge in health liabilities and destroy their health all over again. This illustrates the fact that the ability to adapt and change depends on an individual's personality, and their "true" intentions—who they really are.

CHAPTER 13

Cycles: Can everyone be younger and healthier?

Magic of Life

Magic happens during two instances in human life. These two instances represent the time of infusion and withdrawal of spirit—our birth and death. The birth, we enthusiastically anticipate, while the death, we fearfully dread. We witness what happens to others at these instances, but we never really know what happens to ourselves at these instances. How ironic is that?

We cannot express what happened to ourselves at birth because we don't remember. We cannot share what happened to us at death because we, as we know ourselves, don't exist after death. How these two magical instances are executed is personally unknown to the experiencer, and hasn't been explained by science. As such, the execution of these events is attributed to an unknown entity, God.

Between these two recognizable magical events we live our lives. At the time of birth, when a baby emerges from the mother, the first breath from the outer world is taken. That first breath triggers events within the baby that allow it to live independently from the mother without the umbilical cord. From there, the magic continues as the baby grows each day. Initially, when a baby grows, we're enthusiastic, but this enthusiasm fades as we become adults. We feel invincible in our youth, and that feeling continues until we reach middle age. Around then, our abilities begin to decline, and we become aware of this decline. Along the way, if we happen to acquire a disease, and if the disease threatens our life, we are reminded of the second recognizable magic—death.

In between birth and death, we celebrate life on a yearly basis and call it our birthday. The concept of birthdays introduces the factor of "time" into our aging process. We measure our growth by time, in years. Since time is quantifiable, it's easy to appreciate. Can you imagine just watching someone grow, and not being able to quantify it? It's hard to separate time from the concept of our life because everything in life is measured, expressed, and recorded in time. It's hard to imagine how we would feel and function if we take the concept of time out of our lives. We measure age and maturity by years. Yet, we have all met mature fourteen-year-olds and immature twenty-four-year-olds. This measurement of years is called our chronological age, and chronological age is the normal way to define age in society.

Modern medicine describes the physical growth of a young human and withering of an old human by describing the outward physical characteristics tied to chronological age. Based on this paradigm, we attribute diseases to certain chronological ages. The medical community is surprised when a young person falls ill with an "old person's disease." For example, doctors know that it is unusual for a twenty-three-year-old to have a heart attack. But it does happen. Other examples include diabetes, arthritis, obesity, etc. Because it's hard to study, quantify, and predict how individuals age, we look at it from a population-behavior perspective, and apply statistics to understand that behavior. Based on this method, the majority of the human population is expected to fall into a common pattern of aging, except for a few people who exist outside of this pattern, called "outliers."

No one is able to predict who will follow the common pattern, and who will be an outlier. When an "old person's disease" manifests in a young person, we write it off as an outlier, aberrancy, or bad luck.

We hardly stop to ask, "Could this young person actually be as old as an old person if we take the chronological age out of it?"

Aging is not tied to time. Aging goes on, irrespective of time, and is tied to changes in nature. It is tied to day and night, the sun and the moon, hot and cold, dry and humid, and the changes in seasons. Human civilization conceived the idea of time, and applied that idea to aging, among other things, for practicality. If human beings understood their own nature without the factor of time, we could look past chronology and chronological aging and realize what true living is.

Illusion Revisited

Thinking in terms of chronology is a distraction. Take the example of buying a car. Each model is labeled with a particular year—each car has a "birth year." This enables us to estimate the age of the car from a chronological perspective. However, the birth year of the car doesn't tell us how old the engine really is. A newer car with 80,000 miles may look shiny and nice on the outside, but it doesn't have as much mileage left. On the other hand, an older model with 2,000 miles may have an old design and look withered, but it has plenty of mileage left to drive.

Similarly, how our inner self is aging is not captured or reflected by chronological age. Chronological age is related to the outer self and outer world, but the aging of the inner self is known as *biological aging*. It is the biological age that is directly related to health and disease. It reflects the rate at which our physical, mental, emotional, and spiritual intelligences are aging.

There is a big disconnect between these two forms of aging, and modern medicine does not address this disconnect. I have yet to find a health agency that performs tests to assess biological aging in all of the levels that constitute our inner self (physical, mental, emotional, spiritual, and unknown). This concept is not popularized, and we don't have adequate tools to evaluate all the levels that constitute our inner self.

A person's life span is comprised of cycles of development, or changes, and is defined by their chronological age. These cycles are listed in the table below.

Cycles of development	Chronological age
Pre-natal development	Before birth – Development
Infancy and toddlerhood	0 to 1.5/2 years old – Growth
Early childhood	3 to 5 years old – Growth
Middle childhood	6 to 11 years old – Growth
Adolescence	12 to 18 years old – Growth
Early adulthood	20 to 34 years old – Withering begins
Middle adulthood	35 to 64 years old – Effects of withering manifests
Late adulthood – Young old	65 to 79 years old – Continued withering
Late adulthood – Old old	80 years and older – Continued withering
Death and dying	At any age

Table 13.1: Cycles of human aging.

During the growth period (especially during adolescence and early adulthood), there is a sense of invincibility that pervades us. During this period, we are convinced that we are healthy. This is the illusion of the thirty-year-old we discussed in Chapter 1. It's during this period that most of us begin the unrecognized transition from the Health ("H") quadrant to the Imbalance ("I") quadrant without major symptom manifestation. This period is like the brand-new car that's being driven 20,000+ miles per year. When that happens, the car ages faster, despite being chronologically "young." It is the same for us. Our inner self—whether at the physical level, mental level, emotional level, or spiritual level—can start to age faster, depending on how we live.

Biological aging can be influenced to accelerate or decelerate based on our living habits. More children becoming obese due to poor eating habits or depressed through social media influence are examples of such aging. If the velocity of biological aging exceeds that of our chronological aging, disease begins to settle in (transition to "D" quadrant) at a younger chronological age, and our life span is shortened. According to modern medicine, we "age well" when the velocity of both types of aging are in accord. How about slowing down biological aging to delay development of disease and increase life span? The answer depends on getting rid of the focus on chronological aging and incorporating the idea of biological aging into our concept of health.

The Aging Conundrum

Aging, dying, and death have been a curiosity for scientists for hundreds of years. More recently, the study of aging has become an increasingly focused discipline, generating fields such as anti-aging medicine, regenerative medicine, functional medicine, and metabolic medicine. Nevertheless, it is a field of confusion and controversies. There are several theories for aging, and none have so far proved conclusive. In order to illustrate the amount of work that is being done on this topic, the current evolving theories are illustrated in Figure 13.1 below.

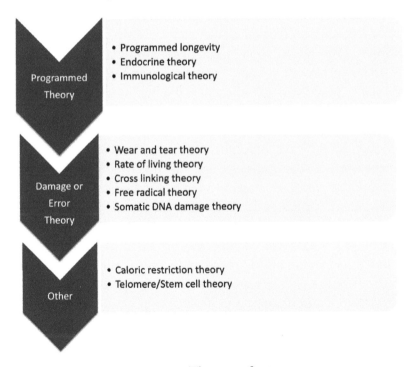

Figure 13.1: Theories of aging.

Rigorous research is ongoing with the goal of achieving human immortality. Until a clear picture emerges out of this scientific exploration, we'll just have to enjoy our immortal superheroes and avatars for the time being. There are a few concepts of aging, however, that are gaining more popularity. These notable theories are the endocrine theory, free radical theory, caloric restriction theory, and stem cell theory. Among these, stem cell theory appears to be the fastest-growing.

In every human being, the magic of life cycles through the phases described in Table 13.1 The early phases are different forms of growth, while the later phases are different forms of withering. Aging typically begins to manifest at the later part of middle adulthood (age 34–65). When the effects of aging start to manifest, it is called senescence.

The predominant perceptible manifestation of aging is the decreasing ability to repair and recover from injuries—meaning a decreased ability to rebalance from an imbalance. The ability to repair and regenerate is highest during the growth phase due to strong health reserve. A wound on a child heals faster than the same wound on an old person. A younger person recovers from alcohol-induced imbalance faster than an old person who ingests the same amount of alcohol.

Compared to the growth phase, the withering phase is characterized by progressive decline in the regenerative capacity of the human body. In essence, as we age, our inner self's ability to renew itself after an insult progressively declines. Since health is the ability to rebalance, our health declines with aging.

It therefore stands to reason that the more we age, the more we have to be actively involved in preserving and renewing our inner self in order to maintain health. Irrespective of this realization, most of us do the opposite. We decrease activities as we age. If we've developed habits that are health assets, this renewal will be easier as we age. If we haven't, the renewal will be harder. This creation of health assets ideally should take place during the growth phase (childhood) or at least during early adulthood (age 20–34 years). If we develop habits that foster a lifestyle of health assets, we will reap the benefits later in life.

It's like putting away money into savings while we are still young. The earlier we start saving, the more return on that investment we have for retirement, and the more post-retirement years we have of financial stability. By creating habits of health assets, and limiting habits of health liabilities, we preserve vital-force of the non-renewable portion, which then acts as our "health savings" to borrow from later in life. Imagine starting to save for retirement at age fifty. Worse still, imagine not even having any savings. The key takeaway is that we should begin developing these healthy habits during childhood and as young adults.

Unfortunately, our children and young adults are not taught this concept. Lack of proper health education across the world robs our children and youth of learning healthy habits. In fact, most of our children and young adults develop habits of health liabilities during their childhood and young adulthood. When the toxic environment around us affects our children, we don't take it seriously, thinking that the young and healthy are able to withstand it—because they are young. That is true, but the toxic environment takes a portion of their future savings, unless they are taught how to renew the lost portion.

Our body is designed to readily withstand a short-time insult, but when the insults become habits, they become liabilities. This predisposes us to rapid biological aging, and subsequently, development of disease.

In the modern era, most chronologically young adults are becoming biologically older than their chronological age. We blame it on factors in the outer world such as an abundance of food, electronics, smoking, alcohol, and recreational drugs. We forget that we have a choice as individuals. It's a matter of controlling the ocean or the sail. Our children are not taught about proper health choices. Their silent partners have the wrong information about health.

The outer world factors mentioned above do not affect our choice, but they greatly influence it due to their convenience. This is one of the reasons chronic diseases like diabetes, obesity, hypertension, anxiety, and depression are beginning to manifest in younger and younger people, including children. Imagine developing diseases during the growth phase where one's ability to repair, regenerate, and rebalance is supposed to be at its peak!

Regeneration and recovery are dependent on renewability. Renewability is about adopting habits that are health assets, resulting in the renewal of our vital-force. We use vital-force to repair and regenerate after an insult. The job of repair and regeneration is carried out by the building blocks of our body—the cells.

The human body begins with the union of two cells—a sperm and an egg. The fertilized egg continues to divide, and makes cells that can differentiate into specialized cell lines to form different organs and tissues. The original, undifferentiated cells have the potential to become any cell line, and are called embryonic stem cells.

Stem cells are naturally segregated, and exist in niche areas of the body in a quiescent stage until called upon. At that point, they become active building blocks to be utilized for the purpose of repair and renewal. These cells behave according to the same concept of renewability of vital-force discussed in Chapter 12.

Stem cells are a great example of the physical form for the concept of the renewable and non-renewable portion of vital-force we have been discussing. For example, those stem cells that are stored in niche areas of the body disengaged and inactive constitute the non-renewable portion. However, the same inactive and disengaged stem cell population has the potential to become any type of cells when needed by any organ or tissue. By transforming, they become actively engaged and gain renewable status. The process and function of stem cells is testament for the concept of non-renewable and renewable vital-forces in us. The vital-force is the same but acquires different status based on engagement and non-engagement.

The problem is that these stem cells decline in number as we age, resulting in less stem cells being available for deployment to repair, regenerate, and rebalance (Figure 13.2). In addition, their function, or ability to transform into any new type of cell, also declines with age (Caplan, 2007).

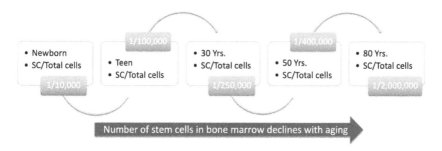

Figure 13.2: Ratio of stem cells to the total number of cells in human bone marrow. SC: Stem Cells.

Descendants of stem cells are called progenitor cells. Progenitor cells divide further and become specialized cells, called effector cells. Aging stem cells have less ability to become progenitor and effector cells compared to young stem cells.

This decline in both number and efficiency of stem cells leads to a reduction in the ability to recover from an insult. As a result, fighting a disease when we're older is like trying to dig a ditch with a serving spoon. Having a reduced ability to recover and rebalance means we're at greater susceptibility for disease and shortened life span. This is not because a disease is lurking but because health is declining. As we age, we must therefore engage in actions that are health assets and reduce actions that are health liabilities. It also helps if we have preserved vital-force from our chronologically younger cycle of life, like putting away money for retirement.

A closer look at stem cells reveals they behave in a programmed and controlled fashion. This behavior is associated with multiple mechanisms in the body, but one especially stands out. The longevity of stem cells appears to be closely related to the protein molecule at the end of our DNA called *telomere* (described in Chapter 11).

Science has discovered that every time a stem cell divides, it uses—and therefore loses—a portion of its telomere. Telomere length has been associated with the longevity of cells; longer telomere equates with longer cell life span and shorter length with short life span. Can this loss of telomere length be minimized?

People who routinely engage in thirty minutes or more of moderate exercise maintain longer telomere length as they age, compared to those that do not exercise. This suggests that regular exercise has a positive influence on telomere length, stem cell number, aging, and health, and that we can influence our own cells through behavioral change.

Vital-force is closely related to biological aging. Chronological aging is a measure of aging, without any useful data in it—meaningless. Remember, aging is the inflation process of health. It takes away our value slowly, over time. Therefore, it makes sense to create strategies that counter this inflation process. We can create a portfolio of actions that are considered health assets to offset the process of biological aging. Every one of us possesses the power to be younger and healthier. The choice is ours to make. A good formula is to *influence the biological aging process and measure the physical manifestation of that process without involving chronological age.*

PART III

HOW DO I DO IT?

8 TRANSFORMATIONAL RULES

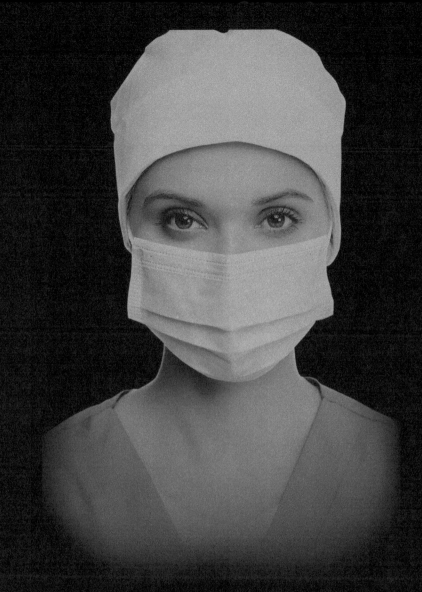

MAKE A COMMITMENT

CREATE YOUR OWN TEAM

GET HEALTHY FROM INSIDE OUT

ENGAGE THE SPIRIT

RECOGNIZE CHANGE DAILY

RENEW HEALTH DAILY

MAINTAIN LIFELONG HEALTH

RECRUIT AN EXPERT ADVOCATE

CHAPTER 14

Rule #1: Make a commitment

Teaching an Old Dog New Tricks

Success in any endeavor depends on the unwavering and continued commitment of the individual to the cause. This can be related to building health, wealth, or even happiness. The degree of commitment depends on the degree of alignment between a logically accepted decision and the preexisting opinion of our silent partner on the issue in question. Usually, an urge to make a resolution and accomplish an outcome emerges at the height of an emotional response to a life event.

The decision by Mr. Cardiologist to look beyond modern medicine to understand health, described in Chapter 3, is such an example. The decisions by Mr. Addict and Mr. Lazy to change their lifestyles so as to be eligible for heart transplant, described in Chapters 7 and 10 respectively, are further examples. They modified their internal dialogue and established a re-alignment between their logical decisions and their silent partners. On the other hand, the cases of Mr. Illusionist (Chapter 1) and Mr. Priest (Chapter 5) had undesirable outcomes because they could not accomplish such an alignment.

The inception for a successful outcome relies on the commitment within an individual to change and adapt. Our thoughts are very powerful because they lead to our words and our actions. Therefore, it's important to be aware of what we tell ourselves. Mahatma Gandhi said, "Watch your thoughts for they become words, watch your words for they become actions, watch your actions for they become habits, watch your habits for they become your character, and watch your character for it becomes your destiny."

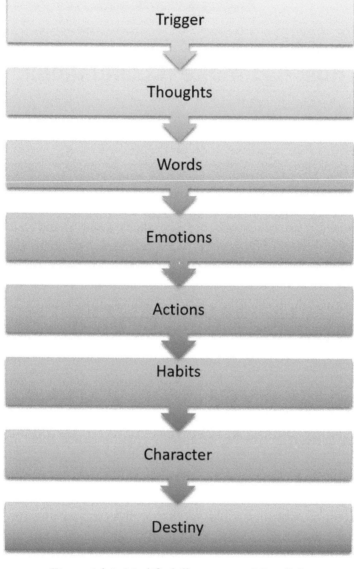

Figure 14.1: Modified illustration of Gandhi's statement on thoughts to destiny.

The first six chapters of this book illustrated different views on health, and the first five of these views are already embedded in our brains. The environment we live in slowly programs these views into us. Just being informed of these wrong views and aware of the correct view is not sufficient for success. We need to do something with that information. As French poet and pioneering aviator, Antoine de Saint-Exupéry once said, "A goal without a plan is just a wish."

After being alerted to the correct view, we have to channel our thoughts, words, and emotions in order to take action. Our thoughts, words, and emotions are powerful attributes, and changing them takes a strong commitment and a plan. By executing that plan (action), we form new, healthy habits. Those healthy habits become a healthy lifestyle—a healthy character. While being healthy is a life-long effort, changing our old patterns of thinking and forming new, healthy patterns takes less than our lifetime. Changing our habits is carried out through a process called neuroplasticity, which was briefly discussed in Chapter 7. In his book, *Psycho-Cybernetics*, the American plastic surgeon, Dr. Maxwell Maltz, described that patients under-going plastic surgery took about twenty-one days to recognize and become accustomed to their new look. He also noted that patients who had an amputation of their limb took about twenty-one days to lose the phantom feeling from their missing limb.

Research conducted at University College London in 2009 reported that the time it takes to form a new brain pattern (new habit) is a range, and not an exact number of days, weeks, or months (Lally, 2010). The majority of the participants in the study formed new habits after around sixty-six days, with a range being 18–254 days. A range with that magnitude suggests that we can't predict, with certainty, how long it will take to form a habit in any individual. This result also attests to the individuality of humans. Each one of us is unique.

While Dr. Maltz's observation of the time taken for habit for-mation is within the range observed by researchers at University College London, individual results vary greatly. One observation is clear: it may take as long as 254 days (approximately eight months) to develop a new habit. However, the journey of 254 days starts with just one day—the first day. It's hard to predict where any one of us will achieve neuroplasticity, but the predictability to maintain our actions until that point is under our control.

Committing to develop a new habit is called "goal intention," and the plan to achieve that goal is "implementation intention." In order to be successful, we must execute both of these intentions and allow enough time for that execution. In healthcare, patients that executed both goal intention and implementation intention were winners. Patients that only had goal intention and failed to execute implementation intention were unsuccessful.

Plenty of people have goal intentions but have no implementation intention. Their failure to execute implementation intention is due to their silent partner's opinion being unaligned with their logical wish for a goal. Their silent partner is a barrier between their goal and the action required to achieve that goal. This is important to recognize when we set a goal. The journey to being healthy begins with the process of retraining our silent partner: getting rid of old, unhealthy ideas and inserting new, healthy ones.

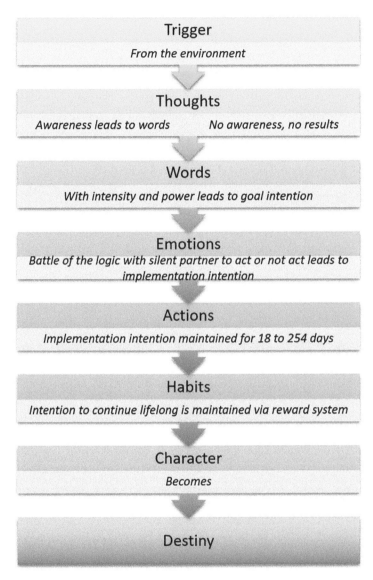

Figure 14.2: Gandhi's concept superimposed with scientific data.

Another important factor is the ability to maintain the implementation intention throughout the journey. Creating a reward system for our inner self accomplishes this. No matter what area the reward is experienced in, the reward should either be measurable and/or recognizable. The reward for physical intelligence could be weight loss, better definition of figure, muscle gain, improved endurance, etc. The reward for mental intelligence could be clarity of thinking, ease of understanding complex concepts, sense of peacefulness, etc. The reward for emotional intelligence could be positive emotions such as joy and happiness, or an improved ability to handle tough emotions without succumbing to them. The reward for spiritual intelligence could be empathy toward others, the ability to maintain neutrality in the face of calamity, etc. Any one of these can act as reward for maintaining our drive toward a desired destiny.

The eight steps described in this part of the book combine the basic ingredients for success. Consider the following as a health code that incorporates these eight steps and our motivation for success:

"I *commit* to a lifestyle of health by creating a *team,* and adopting *self-cleansing* to engage my *spirit* to *recognize, renew,* and *maintain* my health with *guidance.*"

CHAPTER 15

Rule #2: Create your own team

Members

The idea taught in our schools focuses on individual success. Preparing for an exam and working hard to achieve the passing grade in the test without collaboration instills a sense of individuality. If we don't achieve the required grade, we don't progress. We continue to emphasize the notion that success comes from individual effort. Most college graduates are conditioned this way, and continue to exercise this notion in life.

For example, in medical school I was trained to diagnose and treat diseases; I was not trained to be a successful physician. I had no idea how to put together a medical practice and manage the billing, overhead, revenue, expenses, or employees. After medical school, all I had was a certificate informing the world that I had successfully studied diseases. The training during my internship and residency focused on how to become an independent physician and treat those diseases, preparing me further for a one-person show. But today my success depends on working with a team, not just myself.

If we look around, we can see that most things require us to function as part of a team. Raising a family involves a team of parents and children. We have an accountant, a priest, a hairstylist, a manicurist and pedicurist, an automobile mechanic, a grocer, a dry cleaner, a handyman, a plumber, an electrician, etc. We tend to frequent and use the same people over and over again—that is our team for living essentials.

Spirituality is learned and practiced as a team at churches. Companies involve a team of people in different specialties. My institution's heart transplant program's success is due to a team of different professionals that support the process. Successfully getting this book from my desk to your hands was the result of teamwork between author, reviewers, editors, proofreaders, graphic artists, publishers, distributers, and sellers.

It's no different in healthcare. Taking care of a patient requires a team of nurses, medical assistants, phlebotomists, X-ray technicians, cleaners, and physicians. It takes a big team to get a patient through heart transplant, and it's similar in every other medical and surgical specialty. But in addition to an extensive hospital medical team, patients should also have two other types of personal teams to support them. One type of personal team is called the social support team that comes into play during a health crisis. This social support team consists of family members and friends. The importance of such social support team is illustrated by the story of Mr. Supportless.

Mr. Supportless was being admitted to the hospital due to severe heart failure in critical condition. At the time of admission to the hospital, it looked like it was going to be just like any other transplant evaluation. However, it was discovered that he had been denied transplant by other programs due to insufficient social and family support. Mr. Supportless was fully aware of this situation but still did not have enough time to put together a social support team before the health crisis occurred. We identified the lack of social support, and advised him to build a support team in order to qualify for transplant.

After recovering from that hospitalization, it took him about three years to put together such a team, but by then he had become ineligible for transplant because he was no longer in the age window (most transplant programs use a cut-off age of seventy). As a result, he had to settle for the second-best treatment: a mechanical heart pump.

Mr. Supportless shows us the consequences of lacking a social support team. In my experience, I've seen other patients offered only hospice care because of this lack of social support team. Patients that have a very strong social support team have better odds of success when a health crisis occurs. Unfortunately, most people do not realize the importance of a social support team until a health crisis strikes.

Even more important than managing a health crisis is preventing such health crisis. This requires having a team of professionals outside of the hospital system to support maintaining health and prevent disease from setting in. This is accomplished with a team of health professionals—a professional support team. The diagram below illustrates the potential members of a health team for an individual. The individual can choose appropriate members to form their own health team.

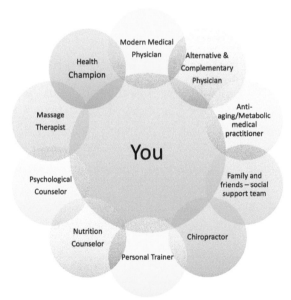

Figure 15.1: Potential members of a health team.

The health team is composed of experts that promote and support the physical, mental, emotional, and spiritual intelligences of an individual. Some of the experts are consultants, others are therapists, and some can do both consultation and treatment. These are experts that one will interact with repeatedly throughout life—similar to how we periodically interact with grocery stores, gas stations, salons, etc. Some of the experts in the team can provide services in multiple aspects. For example, a personal trainer may be additionally certified in yoga and meditation. Some chiropractors are also certified in the use of herbs, supplements, and acupuncture.

Most complementary and alternative medical professionals are trained in multiple modalities, such as anti-aging medicine, acupuncture, functional medicine, herbal therapy, homeopathy, hormone balance, laser therapy, vitamin therapy, etc. Some psychological counselors can also provide life coaching and hypnotherapy.

The services we require to stay healthy will vary from one individual to another, and it's our responsibility to research those services and find the right members for our professional health team, in addition to the social support team of family and friends. This takes time and due diligence.

Understanding Professional Team Members

While I'm a medical practitioner, I'm also trained in the philosophies of acupuncture, yoga therapy, homeopathy, iridology, Ayurveda, and some degree of musculoskeletal manipulation. As such, I'm able to understand the advantages and limitations of these various disciplines to evaluate which ones are better suited, individually or in combination, for a patient's condition.

One cardinal rule is that the purpose of maintaining health is to increase vital-force and slow biological aging in order to prevent the development of disease. If a serious disease develops, however, there is only one place to get treatment—the modern medical system. The healthcare system, with all its inefficiencies, is excellent for emergent disease care.

At the end of the day, when disease appears, most of our personal team members will have less input than the physician. This doesn't mean the team members are useless, but their understanding in the disease space is limited.

In other words, the physician becomes your guide when you have a disease. Why? This is because the majority of the other team members have not seen the inside of a hospital in the same capacity as the medical practitioner, and are not experts in disease care. They are experts in wellness care.

There have been several occasions where I've had heart failure patients come to the hospital at death's door after ignoring modern medicine, and instead trusting only their complementary practitioners. Later, we found out that the complementary practitioners were not even aware that the patient had heart failure. It had been either misdiagnosed or missed entirely. Some of those patients did not survive.

Alternatively, most medical practitioners only pay attention to disease, and ignore the health aspect. An example is that of Mr. Artist discussed in Chapter 3. It's important that both the medical practitioner and the complementary practitioner communicate and collaborate on our health. There should be mutual respect for each other's expertise in their respective fields.

In a team approach to health, the modern physician, complementary physician, anti-aging and metabolic medical practitioner, or our psychological counselor become the frontline guides, while other members may be contacted periodically for support. Most people think in an "either/or" fashion: they have either a modern physician or a complementary physician in their team. They also tend to ignore one or the other practitioner based on what their silent partner tells them. As a result, they miss the substantial benefit of having both in their team.

Attributes of Professional Members

Each member of the team makes a unique contribution to our wellbeing. However, in addition to the unique contribution of their expertise, each team member should also exhibit the following attributes:

- Open-minded to accept a team approach. If they cannot function as a team, it violates the spirit of what we are trying to do.

- Respect for each other's expertise. Lacking respect for other experts infers insecurity in one's own abilities. An insecure person cannot be an asset to us, irrespective of how "good" they are. On the other hand, watch for overconfidence as well.

- Have our best interests in mind while rendering services. If the experts are selling themselves constantly, without recognizing that you have already hired them, it is a warning sign.

- Humble enough to know their own limitations within the sphere of health. Someone who believes they know everything is a liability. Practitioners who know how much they don't know are assets.

- Willing to "stay in their lane" of expertise while giving advice. A tendency to discredit or dismiss other experts' roles is disrespectful to the person who hired them—you.

- Willing to discuss, consult, and collaborate with other experts on your behalf. If no information is communicated, there is no team play.

- They have a team approach to their own health. That tells us that the experts share the same philosophy. If the expert is not aligned with the team health approach philosophy, that expert is a liability.

Remember, the team is supposed to help us become healthy, but you are the captain of this team. It's important that we have a clearly established goal, and build our team with this goal in mind. In the words of Blair Singer, author of *Sales Dogs* and owner of Blair Singer Companies, "One should build a championship team, not a team of champions."

CHAPTER 16

Rule #3: Get healthy from inside out

A Natural Tendency

Every fall, millions of trees shed their leaves only to grow them back the following spring. Trees obey the law of nature based on the seasons. Getting rid of the old and prepare for the new is a form of cleansing. Outwardly, this process of shedding appears to be a loss. It is, in fact, gaining ability. Trees enter dormancy to conserve energy during the winter so that they can bloom again the following spring. Thus, shedding is how trees gain the ability to bloom. There is internal gain in the outward appearance of loss—Yin and Yang.

The concept of cleansing is in alignment with renewability. Renewability is gaining what is lost. Cleansing in health involves getting rid of unwanted substances like toxins in order to preserve and gain energy. All life in nature goes through cyclical cleansing for the purpose of renewal. With regard to trees, shedding leaves during the fall is nature's spontaneous way of renewal process while passing through the four seasons, year after year. Likewise, the human body has a natural tendency to cleanse and renew as we age, called spontaneous cleansing. It is part of healthy living.

The human body performs spontaneous cleansing in many ways. Externally identifiable elimination processes include moving our bowels, urination, sweating, breathing out toxins, tear production in our eyes, secretions of our nose, and the production of wax in our ears. The liver is our most active detox factory.

Examples of internally occurring but externally unidentifiable renewal include cycles of cell production and death in our blood. For example, our red blood cells have a life span of approximately 120 days before they die and new red blood cells are formed. White blood cells, which fight infection, have a variable life span ranging from hours to years. Our platelets have a life span of about nine to twelve days (www.mskcc.org/pe). The blood renews itself by getting rid of old cells and replacing it with new cells. This type of renewal goes on in other organs and tissues as well. Organs and tissues spontaneously get rid of cells in order to accommodate new ones by a process called apoptosis, or programmed cell death. This renewal is inherent to our survival.

This spontaneous process goes on without any additional input from us. In fact, most of us, knowingly or unknowingly, choose a lifestyle that impairs this process, and negatively influences our biological aging. This negative influence accelerates the aging process, and thus the loss of vital-force, leading to a decline in our ability to recover from an imbalance. Eventually, this results in an unhealthy inner self and an environment (Claude Bernard's "Terrain") that can easily be unbalanced—increasing susceptibility to disease and shortened life span.

For most of us, additional cleansing means taking a daily shower and brushing our teeth twice a day (or for some, not even that frequently). As a child, I went through a process, which I perceived at the time, as torture, in a cycle enforced by my parents. All of Saturday is reserved for the process of physical cleansing, separate from the bathing on every other day of the week.

Saturday was the day of the oil bath. First thing in the morning, sesame oil or olive oil (non-synthetic pure oil) was applied and massaged from head to toe. The oil was washed off after allowing a few hours for it to soak in. I was told that this would invigorate the skin's function of protecting the body and elimination of toxins. Oil was applied to the eyes as a method of exercising the tearing mechanism to maintain its integrity.

Once a month, I was given a bitter concoction to be taken on an empty stomach that resulted in diarrhea the entire day. No food, except black tea, is consumed most of that day. This was to facilitate the bowel's absorption and elimination.

Every three months, hydrogen peroxide was administered into both ears to clean the wax that accumulated. A Neti pot was frequently used to clean the nasal passages to promote trapping and eliminating impure materials.

Daily physical exercise was promoted to induce profound sweating and eliminate toxins through the skin. Only the individual performing these rituals can say whether they've achieved the intended result. However, one thing is clear: a philosophy of energizing the body's inherent ability to self-cleanse appears to be a smart thing to do.

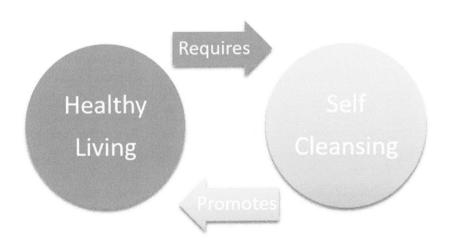

Figure 16.1: Health and self-cleansing are interdependent.

I often contrast those practices of my childhood to what is common practice today. We eat processed and toxic foods in excess, and don't carry out bowel cleansing on a regular basis. Instead, we experience constipation from time to time, and then take chemicals to stimulate the bowels. We breathe polluted air and never once think about cleaning our nasal passages. We smoke, vape, and inhale other toxic materials, causing damage to our lungs. We live sedentary lives and do not promote sweating to eliminate toxins through our skin.

Instead, we take the easy way out and use saunas to sweat, eliminating other additional benefits that exercise provides. Instead of cleaning out the ear canal, we use cotton swabs that actually push the earwax further in. Is this because we are ignorant, or are we simply unmotivated to perform the proper, smarter actions?

Physical Cleanse

Every cell of our body is a unit of our living being. As part of its metabolism, the cell produces waste products in our body. For example, the waste product of cells generating energy is carbon dioxide, which accumulates in the body and leads to an acidic environment unfavorable to cell survival. That's why we eliminate carbon dioxide by breathing it out through the lungs.

Another example of the body's production of toxins is the creation of super-oxides called free radicals. Just as with carbon dioxide, there are internal mechanisms for our body to neutralize and eliminate them. This is the basis of the "free radical theory" discussed in Chapter 13 in relation to biological aging. The remedial agents that take care of free radicals are called antioxidants. As a result, antioxidants are currently promoted as an anti-aging agent.

There are several toxic byproducts that result from our normal processes for living, and the body has respective mechanisms to counter and cleanse itself of each one of them. These internal processes are not obvious to us, but occur 24/7 within our body.

In short, whether we like it or not, we produce toxic waste within ourselves as part of the normal cellular living of our inner self. Fortunately, the body has inbuilt mechanisms to get rid of this toxic waste. If every other variable in our life is unchanged, this ability will stay maintained fairly well, except for the decline through biological aging.

The bad news is that every other variable in our life does not remain the same, which is why there is a need for additional up-keep.

Our activities introduce outer world toxins into our inner self. We eat unnecessary substances that are mixed in with our food to extend its shelf life. Our vegetables and fruits may contain pesticides, while milk and meat contain hormones and antibiotics. Our water and wine may contain heavy metals. We breathe polluted air. We consume beverages and synthetic food that our digestive system and liver don't know what to do with. Additionally, we consume excessively due to easy accessibility and emotional eating.

We apply chemicals to our skin, such as synthetic body lotions, facial make up, and deodorants. These skin products have heavy metals and other materials that are toxic to our cells. Skin absorbs substances it comes into contact with. Anything we put on our skin gets into our body. In modern medicine, administering medications via the skin is a routine process called "transdermal administration." Do you know that the skin is the largest organ in our body? An adult human carries about eight pounds (3.6 kilograms) and twenty-two square feet (2 square meters) of it (*National Geographic*, 2017).

What's more, while it's easily accessible for up-keep, unlike our internal organs, we largely ignore it. With this degree of toxic material entering our inner self, our body's cleansing mechanisms get bogged down. Failure to eliminate these materials results in the accumulation of toxins over time, leading to impaired function of organs and cells.

A need for physical cleansing becomes evident when we consider the level of toxins that accumulate through normal cellular living in addition to environmental pollution. Additionally, if we consider age-related decline in our ability to eliminate these toxins, the case for periodic physical cleansing becomes that much stronger. This periodic self-cleanse should not just facilitate the external elimination mechanisms described above, but also facilitate the internal elimination mechanisms of our body.

Detox programs influence the internal elimination mechanisms of our bodies. There are several programs, and choosing the most suitable for us is a process of trial and error. Three members of our team can help with recommendations: the modern medical practitioner, the complementary/alternative medical practitioner, and the anti-aging medical practitioner. However, as a general rule, a cleanse program should deliver at least the following benefits:

- Consist of natural, organic, and non-synthetic nutrients.
- Simultaneously deliver essential and healthy nutrients while eliminating toxins. These nutrients should have been obtained and produced from original food sources without any extra processing.
- Last long enough to influence a change in habits based on what we discussed in Chapter 14 about modifying our silent partner through neuroplasticity.
- Make us feel more energetic by promoting good sleep, appetite, and endurance.
- Eliminate emotional eating habits.
- Change the way we react to our own emotions.
- Facilitate weight management.
- Have a lasting transformational influence in our lifestyle by influencing other levels of our inner self, too (Figure 16.2).

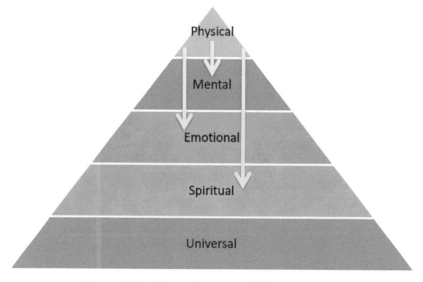

Figure 16.2: The influences of physical cleanse on other beings of our inner self.

Realize that these benefits may take more than the minimum duration recommended by the detox program. Individual results vary, and identifying the right product takes trial and error, or can come from a trusted source.

Emotional Cleanse

Just like the liver is our major detox organ for toxic physical agents and materials, the brain is the major processing center of our mental and emotional activities. Facilitating the cleansing mechanisms of our inner self includes the physical, mental, emotional, and spiritual levels and their corresponding intelligences.

We live in a world of constant, and in my opinion, excessive sensory input, that constantly influence all levels of our inner self. Some of the inputs are positive, some are negative, and others are neutral. The net input tends to be negative. As discussed previously, any input received is quickly assessed, and a response is generated based on our personal logic and the judgment of our silent partner.

When those are in conflict, our social self (ego) doesn't know how to manifest, and the conflict continues until it's directly addressed and resolved. This constant existence of conflicts uses our vital-force, and thus drains life-flow, leading to a decline in our ability to maintain balance—health. It is like having a crossed wire leading to a short circuit in the electrical system resulting in undetected slow drain in electricity. We may not notice it at the beginning, until the electrical bill goes up. If unaddressed and gets worse over time, it can even start a fire. It's the same in health; vital-force depletion may not be recognized until a disease develops.

In addition to draining vital-force, these mental and emotional conflicts also cloud our judgment. These conflicts are unnecessary, toxic, and result in underperformance at all levels of the inner self, as well as the corresponding intelligences.

Consider a trigger, either at home or work, which caused you to be angry. That emotion—anger—needs an outlet because it is energy in motion. We want to do something about that anger, but may be unable to come up with a socially acceptable response. At this point, there is conflict between our emotional intelligence and silent partner.

Every conflict is associated with an emotion whether we recognize it or not. This emotional conflict lives in us forever unless we address it and come up with a resolution. When unattended, this emotional conflict continues to drain vital-force further affecting our thinking and actions.

A good example of this is a child getting upset for not getting what they want. They act out by being moody, refusing to go to school, or ignoring parents until the conflict is resolved. After a while, children forget about it, resolve it within themselves by bargaining for something else, and move on. But if the conflict is strong, it may not get resolved, and they may take it further. Imagine someone taking it to the next level resulting in underperformance or unusual behavior at school, work, or home—we are all aware of individuals in whom childhood conflicts continue to live during adulthood. In adulthood, these thinking processes and actions are generated based on the initial conflict that occurred during childhood, and are toxic to us.

In the end, all of this boils down to one single question: will a trigger, internal or external, result in a transformational outcome or in an emotional conflict? This depends on our response to that trigger. Consider the simple formula below:

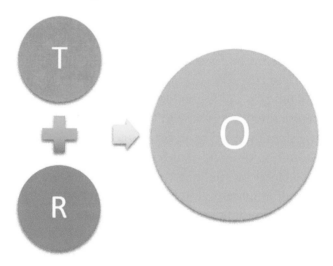

Figure 16.3: T = environmental trigger; R = our response to trigger; O = ultimate outcome.

Whether the outcome is favorable or not depends largely on our response, not the trigger. If the outcome is unfavorable, trigger is not to be blamed, our response is. Most people are not adequately equipped to properly respond to these triggers. There is a tendency to address and correct the trigger instead of changing how *we* respond to it. As a result, we don't always create the desired outcome. In Mahatma Gandhi's words, "If you want to change the world, change yourself and the world will change itself."

The ability to respond in a way that creates a favorable outcome involves use of "coping mechanisms." Coping skills don't come from outside, but rather from within. Coping skills, however, are learned methods. Not everyone learns beneficial coping skills. Coping skills relate to one's ability to resolve conflicts between the logical drive and the drive of the silent partner. The stronger drive will win.

Usually, our silent partner determines the response to a trigger, and thus the outcome. Looking back at Mr. Addict's (Chapter 7) and Mr. Lazy's (Chapter 9) initial struggles and subsequent success illustrates the difficulties they had with this aspect. Their initial lack of coping skills in the face of a life-threatening disease resulted in passive-aggressiveness and non-compliance. But after modifying their silent partner, they were able to create a favorable outcome. Mr. Priest (Chapter 7) on the other hand, did not commit to modifying his silent partner, and it cost him his life.

The silent partner's response to a trigger is rapid and reflexive. Because we are so used to agreeing with the silent partner, we don't recognize its involvement in these reflexes—it is second nature to us. As a result, conflicts accumulate within us and become our unwanted, negative baggage. The burden of this baggage prohibits optimal functioning and drains vital-force, leading to negative life-flow and ill-health. Scientists are beginning to discover the importance of personality traits in the development of disease, as well as disease-outcome.

Just as we must cleanse our physical bodies of toxins, we must also cleanse our toxic emotions. A case is then made for what I call *emotional cleansing*. Emotional cleansing essentially refers to conflict resolution. This applies not just to recent conflicts, but also to old conflicts that are buried deep within us. Some may have been embedded in our childhood and teenage years. In addition to draining vital-force, they also influence our decision-making ability by introducing bias. Imagine the power of the mental, emotional, and spiritual intelligences, if we could free up more of the vital-force trapped by deep-seated conflicts. Emotional cleansing has the ability to free up that power (Figure 16.4).

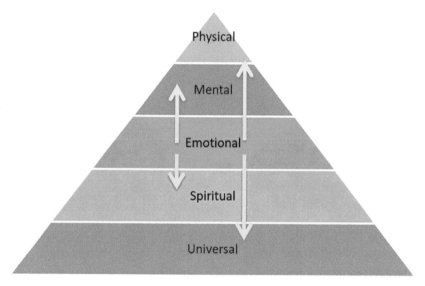

Figure 16.4: The influences of emotional cleanse
on other beings of our inner self.

Many people get offended when psychological counseling is recommended to unload the baggage of conflicts within them. This is because they falsely believe that psychological counseling is for people with mental illness. That is a myth. In fact, we all need psychological counseling to prevent these conflicts from impairing us because our environment is increasingly becoming emotionally polluted. There is nothing wrong with getting help to deal with conflicts, and learning skills for effective conflict resolution. Remember: the psychological counselor is part of our health team.

Most of us are quite skilled at resolving surface conflicts, and some conflicts can be resolved by consulting our friends, peers, mentors, parents, siblings, etc. However, deeper conflicts that cannot be solved by these means may require professional help.

In such circumstances, we must admit to ourselves that the conflict requires professional counseling for resolution. In which case, the following rules may optimize the outcome:

- The counselor should be trained in the area of counseling required.
- The counselor should not be someone known to us, therefore, eliminating bias.
- The counselor should be paid for their services. In Robert Kiyosaki's words, "Free advice is the worst advice one can get."
- We should be willing to accept feedback that we may not want to hear, and be prepared to receive other views and opposing opinions.
- Identification of the correct counselor may take trial and error.
- We should be open and honest with our innermost feelings while communicating with the counselor. Patient-client confidentiality laws bind licensed counselors, prohibiting disclosure of our personal information.
- If a counselor is not for you for the right reasons (not because they are telling you what you don't want to hear), do not feel obliged to continue.
- We should be willing to perform the exercises recommended by the counselor and dedicate time for change. Remember, retraining our silent partner takes time (approximately 18 to 254 days) and effort.

In the BMIT, the emotional level is placed right in the middle, separating the physical and mental levels from the spiritual and universal levels. The emotional plane is a very powerful plane; this intelligence has the power to either make us (if handled right) or break us (if handled wrong).

CHAPTER 17

Rule #4: Engage the spirit

The Real Deal

Human spirit is the fountain of youth, and vital-force emanates from that spirit creating life-flow, which animates the human body. Infusion of vital-force enables the life-flow to maintain the balance of our inner self, giving us the ability called health. As vital-force is spent, life-flow diminishes, and human animation declines. This natural decline manifests through the speed of biological aging. In the background of biological aging, adopting habits of health liabilities further depletes available vital-force leading to internal imbalance and even development of disease.

Chapter 5 discussed how to understand health from the point of view of the human spirit, while Chapter 8 covered the evidence for the spirit and its involvement in health. In Chapter 8, we also discussed that the spirit and the body are two separate entities that co-exist, evidenced by the unusual effects of organ transplant.

Our success in health depends on how skilled we are in maintaining the body-mind union. This continued maintenance requires engaging our spirit, and our success in health depends on how skilled we are in this endeavor. Without that engagement, the health of the body cannot be maintained for long.

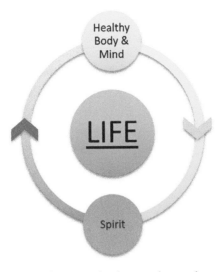

Figure 17.1: The spirit-body-mind interdependence.

Spirit animates the body and mind and uses our brain to process the product of that animation so that the product can be expressed to the outer world. The body/mind combination in turn requires spirit for animated function; body, mind, and spirit are dependent on each other. This animation and manifestation relates to the five levels of our inner self. The physical level refers to the body and its organs. The mental, emotional, spiritual, and the universal levels refer to the mind. The organ brain at the physical level is the processing center for the mind to finally express itself to the outer world. The spirit can animate our body without manifesting to the outer world, like a person in a disease related or medically induced coma—it's just that the outer world cannot perceive the animated intelligences of that spirit, because the processing center (the brain) is out of commission. A functional body and mind is required for processing and expressing the five manifestations of the spirit (physical, mental, emotional, spiritual, and universal).

Letting Go of Our Inner Self

As seen, spirit underlies the manifestation of the five components of inner self. During that manifestation, our spirit animates the physical, mental, emotional, and spiritual intelligences. As a result, our attention is directed at these four intelligences. But—the spirit exists at the unknown/universal level. To engage it, we need to transcend the four levels that the spirit animates.

The spirit is our true presence, but it's masked by the other four intelligences like how smoke can mask a fire. When our attention is captured by one of the other four intelligences, our attention lingers there, but never transcends to its origin. We don't connect with the spirit. As a result, we deny spirit the opportunity to engage us in our daily activities.

The spirit is always waiting to be engaged; our attention just doesn't get to that level. Training our attention to transcend beyond the manifestations (smoke) of the spirit creates the possibility of being one with the spirit (fire). Success is achieved when the spirit is engaged and aligned with our actions.

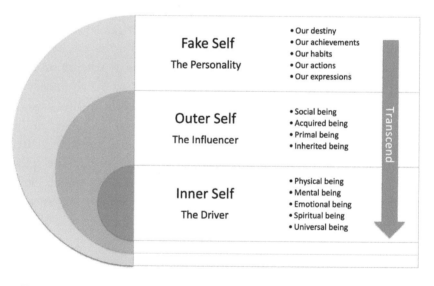

Figure 17.2: Transcending the fake self and outer self to the inner self.

At the first occurrence of the magic of life—when an infant is born—the body is united with the first breath and the spirit is engaged. At that time, there are only two outward manifestations that exist: the physical body and its primal self. All that exists in the baby at this time is the innocence of the body and the universal/unknown level—the primal self and spirit. Subsequently, as we go through childhood, we continue developing and nurturing additional layers (intelligences) of our being and begin to identify ourselves through those manifestations (Figure 17.2). Additionally, living in a society requires us to generate our acquired being—silent partner—that enables socially acceptable behavior.

The secret to re-engaging the spirit is to learn to disengage from the barriers that stand between our attention and our spirit. These barriers include our fake self (personality), outer self, and the four intelligences of the inner self (all except the final levelthe universal level). *It's like becoming an infant again to realize the power and innocence of the sprit.*

When I was first introduced to meditation and yoga, my answer to the guru's question, "Who are you?" was related to my personality (fake self), and not my real being. The guru's intention was to alert me to the possibility of another presence within—the spirit. Yoga is the only discipline that I found effective in helping transcend the barriers that stand between our attention and spirit.

The traditional yoga consists of eight limbs of practice. The regular practice of eight limbs of yoga leads to super-consciousness or reaching one's own spirit to become one with the universal intelligence. As one can see, meditation and yoga exercises are two of the eight limbs as detailed below.

Limb 1: Restrains—the five moral injunctions.
Limb 2: Observances—fostering the five positive qualities.
Limb 3: Postures—physical yoga exercises.
Limb 4: Regulation of breath—yogic breathing.
Limb 5: Drawing the senses inward to still the mind—preparation for concentration.
Limb 6: Concentration—focusing on a single object.
Limb 7: Meditation—transcending the levels of inner self.
Limb 8: Super-consciousness—becoming one with the universal intelligence.

(Recommended reading: *The Sivananda Companion to Yoga*; Simon & Schuster.)

Meditation – Tool for Engaging Our Spirit

For centuries, meditation has been advocated as a means to self-realization. Buddha described self-enquiry as peeling the layers of an onion. The practice of meditation facilitates this by transcending the layers of fake self, outer self, and the intelligences of the inner self. Frequent meditation creates a pathway to engage the spirit by training us to let go of the components of our fake self. Meditation is the practice of doing nothing, and thus allowing for the spontaneous manifestation of the spirit. Consider the steps of meditation below:

> **Step 1.** Choose a quiet place to sit alone—this minimizes the external triggers of the outer world from activating our intelligences. *This is outer world withdrawal.*

> **Step 2.** Withdraw the attention from the outer world and fake self, and focus internally upon the inner self—this accomplishes the release of the outer self. *This is withdrawal of outer self.* At this time we are left with our inner self only (Figure 17.3).

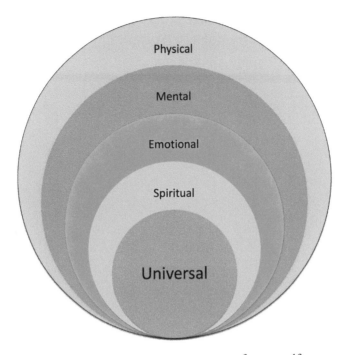

Figure 17.3: Active components of inner self
at the beginning of meditation.

Step 3. Sit quietly, unmoving. Close your eyes, and feel your breath—this accomplishes the release of physical intelligence. *This is sensory withdrawal.*

Step 4. Focus your attention on your breath, a word, or a mantra—this accomplishes the release of mental intelligence by numbing the brain. *This is mental withdrawal.*

Step 5. While observing your breath or repeating a mantra, if a thought arises, let go of the thought and continue to focus on your breath or mantra—this accomplishes the disengagement of the emotional intelligence from thoughts. *This is emotional withdrawal.* At this time we are left with only the two deeper components of our inner self—the real deal (Figure 17.4).

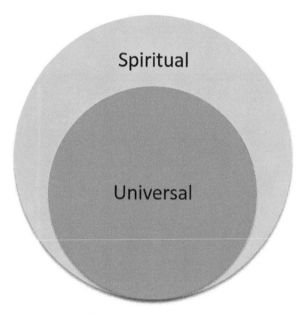

Figure 17.4: Active components of inner self accessed deep into meditation.

Step 6. Continue to repeat steps 4 & 5.

By repeatedly training ourselves to let go of the intelligences that are processed through our brain, we eliminate them from engaging our attention. Over time, this training of repeated disengagement frees our attention to engage the spirit that resides at the deepest level.

Yoga Exercises – A Tool for Permeating the Spirit Throughout the Body

Ancient Hindus understood the importance of allowing the spirit of the universal intelligence (universal level) to permeate the other four intelligences, thus uniting all levels of the inner self. We've seen through previous chapters that human health requires a balance not only within a single level of existence, but between all levels of existence.

The Sanskrit word *yoga* means "union of body and mind." In other words, engaging the spirit with the other intelligences of our inner self. In regard to the BMIT, yoga means uniting the universal level with the physical, mental, emotional, and spiritual levels, thus allowing permeation of our spirit into the other four intelligences.

Contrast the idea of yoga exercises with the idea of meditation. Meditation is withdrawal of all intelligences in order to engage our attention with the spirit. Yoga exercise is re-engagement of those withdrawn intelligences with the attention that is now focused on the spirit.

> **Step 1.** Choose the same time of day to practice yoga and find a quiet place with all electronics turned off and put away. *This is withdrawal of outer world triggers.*

> **Step 2.** Perform exercises with the attention on delicately combining the breath with the movements of the postures, and maintain that focus. *This is re-engagement of the physical intelligence with the spirit.*

> **Step 3.** Continue to hold the posture and maintain that focus. *This is re-engagement of the mental intelligence with the spirit.*

> **Step 4.** Feel the emotions generated by the comfort/discomfort of the physical body that pass through your mind while the posture is held. Overcome your emotions and continue practicing the posture. *This is re-engagement of the emotional intelligence with the spirit.*

Through this, we can see that yoga exercise is, in fact, *meditation in motion*. Unfortunately, this concept is lost to modern yoga teaching and practice. Most yoga is currently practiced as mere physical exercise. The old scriptures suggest performing meditation first, followed by hatha yoga exercises to enhance this disengagement/engagement cycle. This trains our attention to first contact the spirit, and then allows it to permeate our inner self.

It is extremely important to choose how and where you learn these practices, and who teaches you. Failure may result not because we don't know the exercises, but because we aren't taught the right intention behind the practice. There is no shortcut to, or modification of, the right intention.

Both meditation and yoga require withdrawal from the outer world and fake self, as that step enhances our ability to contact our outer and inner self. The idea is that our inner and outer self generates our fake self to manifest in the outer world. Transcending the fake self is the first step in order to reach the other selves.

There are many practices to engage the spirit and allow it to permeate the other intelligences, but none surpass the sophistication of meditation and yoga.

CHAPTER 18

Rule #5: Recognize change daily

The 3R Formula

Awareness is the first step in recognizing a change in our health status, as seen through the HIDE quadrants discussed in Chapter 10. It's easy to identify when you shift into the Disease ("D") quadrant, however, the most important shift we want to recognize and promptly rectify is the shift from the Health ("H") quadrant to the Imbalance ("I") quadrant.

In order to recognize the shift through quadrants, we must be aware of items capable of being precisely identified or realized by the mind, or in other words tangible, so that a change from baseline can be recognized. The formula for accomplishing this is the 3R process: recognize, rebalance, and remain balanced.

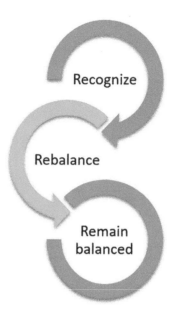

Figure 18.1: Illustration of the 3R formula for monitoring and correcting transitions in health.

Once the first step of the 3R process is achieved, it is easy to adopt or devise methods to rebalance and continue those efforts to remain in balance. Keeping in line with the understanding of the BMIT (Body-Mind Interaction Triangle), every level of the triangle needs to be balanced. Therefore, we need to be aware of the tangible manifestations of each level in order to recognize changes.

The characteristics described in this chapter serve as elements that can be monitored daily to recognize changes in life-flow. A total of nineteen perceivable manifestations of each level are illustrated in Figure 18.2 and are described in this chapter.

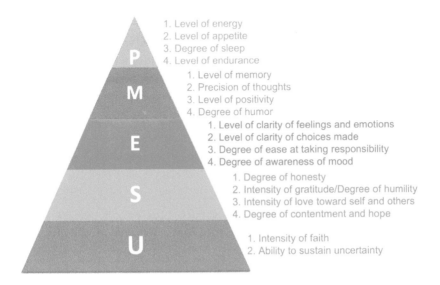

Figure 18.2: P=Physical; M=Mental;
E=Emotional; S=Spiritual; U=Universal

At the Physical Level

Physical level is what we are most familiar with. Our five sensory organs process the sensations generated by the appropriate triggers; vision, sound, smell, taste, and touch. Therefore, sensations and the resulting physical actions are the manifestation of this level. Sensations are the means by which communication is input into our physical intelligence at this level. Our physical intelligence in turn, communicates to us mainly via alterations in the four manifestations described below.

1. Level of Energy

This usually manifests as our willingness to take on the day. For example, do you start worrying on Sunday about Monday? Do you wake up in the morning and feel too sluggish to carry out your responsibilities? Do you hear yourself frequently say, "This is too much," or "I can't go on," etc.? Do you want to postpone your exercise routine to the next day? If we hear ourselves say these or similar statements, there is an imbalance at the level of physical intelligence and it is beginning to drain vital-force, resulting in a decline in life-flow.

When such indication of vital-force imbalance occurs, the worst thing we can do is ignore it, but most people do just that. They drink coffee, or some other caffeinated beverage, to mask the feeling, but this ignores the root cause of the imbalance, and allows for its continuation.

What these sensations tell us is that we are in the Imbalance ("I") quadrant, and should not allow the imbalance to persist. Persisting means we will soon be shifting toward the Disbalance ("D") quadrant. Low physical energy and mental/emotional energy are inter-related; therefore, our next step should be to look at the mental/emotional level.

2. Level of Appetite

I want to elaborate a little bit on how our society has changed when it comes to food-related appetite. First, we consume food based on time of day rather than the body's hunger signal. We do this for several reasons such as work, scheduled lunch breaks, lack of time for breakfast, and easy availability of food in industrialized countries. Even children often are fed their evening meals based on their extra-curricular activity, which could sometimes lead to them being fed before they get hungry. If food consumption occurs before hunger develops, opportunity to monitor the level of our appetite for food is lost.

Another instance where we do not allow hunger as an indication to consume food is during emotional eating. Overwhelming emotions have a tendency to automatically trigger a propensity for comfort food. This action is a coping mechanism. We have been trained in this fashion from our infancy. When a baby cries, it either gets a pacifier, a bottle of milk, or its mother's breast—all related to the mouth. The baby may not be crying out of hunger, but nevertheless, the first attempt to console the baby is oral in nature. We're therefore trained to fill the mouth during any imbalance or conflict, irrespective of whether the issue is physical, mental, emotional, or spiritual.

Most Eastern disciplines advocate fasting to fight illness. Doctors inquire about appetite on a daily basis when patients are hospitalized, yet, during the normal course of the day, we hardly pay attention to it. In addition, one also wants to pay attention to one's appetite in other means, such as appetite for life, new experiences, knowledge, and sex. All of these can be blunted when the body begins to shift toward an unbalanced state.

3. Degree of Sleep

Altered quality of sleep is another signal that our body gives us when it shifts toward an imbalanced state. Sleep is also another natural renewal function that is affected early, when the body's equilibrium begins to change. This is the time the body is able to restore and replenish the energy that has been used during the day. Normally, in a balanced state ("H" quadrant), one should be able to achieve the following with sleep:

- Fall asleep within five to ten minutes of lying down without sleep aids.
- Have minimal disturbance during sleep such as tossing and turning, snoring, etc.
- Sleep an adequate amount of time for full restoration (see table below).
- Wake up in the morning without an alarm clock with full energy and a clear head.
- Not remember too many dreams.

It is important to know how much sleep one needs, and it's important to monitor the quality and duration of sleep that we get. A chart with the recommended amount of sleep is given below for reference.

Age	Duration of sleep
0 - 3 months (newborn)	14 - 17 hours
4 - 11 months (infant)	12 - 15 hours
1 - 2 years (toddler)	11 - 14 hours
3 - 5 years (pre-school)	10 - 13 hours
6 – 13 years (school age)	9 – 11 hours
14 - 17 years (teen)	8 – 10 hours
18 - 25 (young adult)	7 – 9 hours
26 - 64 (adult)	7 - 9 hours
65 and above (older adult)	7 - 8 hours

Table 18.1: Sleep duration recommendations by the National Sleep Foundation based on age.

4. Level of Endurance

It is normal to feel fatigued or tired at the end of the day, but if there is fatigue at any other time, particularly without a hard day of work (physical, mental, or emotional), then it is abnormal. Explore the underlying reason or seek help. Most common and under-recognized reasons for fatigue are dehydration, lack of restorative sleep, lack of vitamins and minerals in our diet, and hormone imbalances. If these issues are not present, it is time to check for disease.

Endurance level is directly tied to vital-force, therefore when one is in imbalance, the body struggles to supply the needed energy to accomplish normal tasks. This implies significant biological aging, or the presence of imbalance or disease.

At the Mental Level

Feelings, thoughts, and intellectual activity are the manifestations of this level. The mental intelligence connects to us through our thoughts, and we connect back to it by reflecting on those thoughts.

1. Level of Memory

As soon as we wake up, our memory becomes actively engaged. We often take this for granted. Vividly remembering what we have said and done in the distant past, as well as just a few minutes ago, is crucial to our functioning, and it's affected when we are in an unbalanced state.

It is important to recognize any changes in how we remember things. Memory is carried out by several parts of the brain working together; it is not stored in one part. An imbalanced state affects how the brain's synchronizations are carried out, and results in defects in our memory.

If there is a change in this function, we need to stop and reflect on the reasons for this, and correct it immediately. If we forgot where we put our car keys and are repeatedly spending time looking for them, we may want to take a moment to stop and reassess the state of our inner balance.

2. Precision of Thoughts

Precision refers to our ability to make split-second decisions and carry them out. It also relates to the clarity of our thoughts. We need to have a sound nervous system as well as a sound body-mind interaction with balanced vital-force in order to have precision of thoughts. If we find ourselves lacking this precision, our body may not be as balanced as it could be.

Usual indicators are incidents such as saying the wrong things, dropping things, knocking things over, absentmindedness, and even scratching your front wheels on the curb while parking. These are indicators of abnormal integration of the nervous system and body-mind connection. Abnormal integration is a result of an unbalanced state of the person and their vital-force.

3. Level of Positivity

Every day we don't feel positive, that is an indication our system is not in balance. People who are in a balanced state are full of energy, light on their feet, and have a positive attitude with regard to their day and life. Feeling negative about our surroundings, events, and life in general is an indication of an unbalanced state. This means that we are internally fighting a conflict. It is important not to ignore this state, nor give excuses such as having too much work, or someone else didn't do their job, etc. If that is true, then it is time to realize that those factors are unbalancing us, and take action to rebalance.

At the end of the day, even if it's someone else or the environment that made us feel unbalanced, it is us who are going to sustain the imbalance. Positivity breeds positivity. It renews our energy, while excessive and prolonged negativity depletes it.

4. Degree of Humor

I find that most people (myself included) don't feel humor on a regular basis. There are days that I feel very light, and I joke with people around me, and yet there are other days when I'm very serious, and I don't even smile when greeting others. This bothers me. For me, it is an indication of the imbalance within myself.

The ability to connect with others is the first requirement for humor. If this is absent, humor does not exist. Being positive, feeling good about ourselves, feeling genuinely cheerful, and looking at the "good side of things" are important requirements for humor.

Therefore, the presence of humor presupposes the presence of these factors. If we monitor our level of humor, then we are monitoring these underlying requirements that tell us about our state of balance. Aspects of humor are lost when excessive emotions are experienced or perpetuated.

For example, if we are angry, it is hard to crack a joke, or even appreciate a joke. Anger, in Chinese medicine, is considered a result of imbalance in a complex collection of bodily functions described as the "liver." As a result, lack of humor from anger can be an indication of an imbalance of the "liver" in Chinese medicine. The concept of "liver" in Chinese medicine does not exactly correlate with the actual organ liver that we understand from human anatomy. This appears to be a simple example. However, oftentimes, we explain our lack of humor by identifying an existing mental or emotional state such as anger and may not even realize the presence of an additional deeper layer of imbalance described above. The key to reversing such state depends on how clearly we identify the original imbalances that lie deep within us.

At the Emotional Level

Emotions and biological reactions triggered by those emotions are manifestations of this level. The emotional intelligence processes these emotions and communicates with us through biological reactions and impulses. The emotions and biological reactions collectively lead to recognizable impulses at conscious level. Recognizable impulses lead to actions. Therefore, we, in turn, respond to this level by performing an action arising out of these impulses. The actions we choose to respond with depend on our coping mechanism.

1. Level of Clarity of Feelings and Emotions

This refers to the precise understanding of our own feelings, as they are experienced. In order to be precise about the feelings elicited inside us, we need to be aware of the vocabulary that describes different feelings. Feelings are sensations that are perceived at mental level for more than a few seconds. Feelings should have a time component and an intensity component in order to reach the threshold to elicit our awareness of them at the mental level. In other words, they should be present for a certain time at certain strength for us to become aware of them. We don't become aware of weak and fleeting sensations as they lack the intensity and time components. Strong feelings, when perpetuated, over minutes to hours, become emotions and elicit biological reactions within our body. Fight or flight reaction produced by the emotion "fear" is such an example of a biological reaction. In this instance, our heart rate and blood pressure increases in anticipation of the action of either fleeing the scene or fighting the adversary. Emotions, therefore, produce actions through biological reactions within us irrespective of whether an external physical action is carried out or not. These actions can be either a health asset or a health liability. And emotions, when stronger and perpetuated over hours, days, weeks, and months, along with the accompanying biological reactions, become mood. Mood, therefore, is an emotion and its associated biological reaction perpetuated over a long period of time. As a result, a mood can therefore be a health asset or a liability.

In common conversations, however, we use feelings, emotions, and mood synonymously. Such synonymous use clouds the understanding of what is being felt and prevents clarity. Therefore, giving a proper vocabulary and duration to what is being felt will help precise recognition of the experience. A full account of emotions is beyond the scope of this book. However, prominent psychologist and author, Robert Plutchik's description of basic emotions and their derivative emotions are described below:

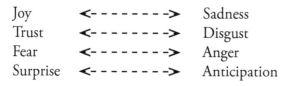

There are several descriptions of emotions with different combinations based on the leading psychologists who proposed them. However, a general consensus exists. This is one version. It is proposed that these basic emotions give rise to other emotions when they exist together.

Joy + Trust = Love (opposite is Remorse)
Joy + Anticipation = Optimism (opposite is Disapproval)
Fear + Trust = Submission (opposite is Contempt)
Fear + Surprise = Awe (opposite is Aggression)
Surprise + Sadness = Disapproval (opposite is Optimism)
Sadness + Disgust = Remorse (opposite is Love)
Anger + Disgust = Contempt (opposite is Submission)
Anger + Anticipation = Aggressiveness (opposite is Awe)

The above set of emotions makes us realize the lack of vocabulary that we possess for the multitude of emotions that we experience on a daily basis. I recommend that one familiarize themselves with the definitions of at least the emotions included here. There are other combinations that result in other emotions and can be learned, but they are beyond the scope of this book.

It is normal to feel emotions, and it's important to recognize when they are perpetuated. Any perpetuated emotion in excess leads to imbalance by stealing vital-force energy, irrespective of whether they are positive or negative.

2. Level of Clarity of Choices Made

If we are clear about our choices, we are in balance. If we are not clear, or we are uncertain, our balance is disrupted. It is important to pay attention to this aspect during our daily activities, including our choices with regard to food, alcohol, fun, relationships, workflow, etc.

In fact, clarity of our choice depends on our clarity of emotion and mood. The right coping mechanism to an emotional trigger is important, so we should monitor the choices we make. If we choose to embark on health liabilities, our choice indicates that we are not in a balanced state. If we have difficulty with coping mechanisms in response to a stressful trigger, we should seek help from a mentor or a psychological counselor.

3. Degree of Ease at Taking Responsibility

How easy is it for us to take responsibility not just for achievements, but also for failures, mistakes, and faults? This does not mean that we simply apologize and move on. It means that we take full responsibility and make corrective action. An apology with the intention to remedy the situation is not a sign of weakness, but an empty apology is, whereas the ability to think clearly and take responsibility is a manifestation of balance.

If we are unable to do this, or if we feel reluctant, we should look within for imbalances. Eastern philosophies tell us that we have the power to make our lives just the way we want them to be. It follows that if we create a mess, health-wise or otherwise, we take responsibility, and there is no reason to feel guilty about it. Rather, start corrective measures.

4. Degree of Awareness of Mood

I have alluded to mood under clarity of feelings and emotions above. Mood is easy to recognize because it lingers around for a while. What's important to recognize is not the mood itself but the shift between moods. For example, have you ever felt that your mood level goes down when you see someone being insulted or hurt? On the other hand, have you ever felt that your mood level goes up when you witness an "act of good" being performed? These are examples of a shift in our mood compared to the mood that existed prior to witnessing either of these events. The emotions elicited by these events may be fear and anger (negative feelings) with regard to the first example, and joy and surprise (positive feelings) with regard to the second. It is important to recognize that the shift will be immediately recognized as a feeling or emotion due to the time component in defining the experience and becomes mood when stronger in intensity and lingers for a prolonged period of time.

As a result, positive feelings and actions elevate our mood level, while negative ones lower our mood level. Similarly, meditation and "quiet time" result in minimizing our tendency to become attached to moods. Mood is actually an easy parameter to monitor with regard to our emotional level of functioning. Learning how to exercise this in our daily life leads to tangible benefits.

At the Spiritual Level

We are now embarking to the deeper levels of human functioning and the comprehension gets complex. The spiritual intelligence connects to us through unexplainable feelings. In other words, we get an impulse, but we don't know where it comes from or what triggered it. It is like getting a sudden "notion." We cannot fully define what is being felt. It is vague. If we spontaneously feel this way, usually, it is a result of the spiritual level trying to communicate with us. We engage with this level through hope and trust. While the communication from this level can be difficult to appreciate, the following five derivatives of this level are easily identifiable.

1. Degree of Honesty

Honesty requires transcending our physical, mental, and emotional intelligences, as it is deeper than these levels. Thus, it requires courage, balance, and a tremendous amount of self-confidence. When I say honesty, I do not mean simply stating what comes to mind—discretion and tact are necessary. Most importantly, honesty requires us to be honest with ourselves first, and honest with others second.

Being honest with ourselves and others means that we are balanced and have a strong physical, mental, and emotional level of functioning. If we find the need to lie, then it is time to take a good look at the status of our spiritual level, as well as the other levels above it.

2. Intensity of Gratitude

Being able to appreciate the good things in life and being grateful for receiving them are signs of a healthy mind and spirit, and by extension, vital-force. When we are well-balanced, everything appears magnificent and admirable, and out of admiration comes gratitude. The intensity of gratitude we feel should be monitored on a daily basis. If it is lacking, we are not well-balanced at the spiritual level. On the other hand, practicing gratitude helps balance our inner self.

3. Degree of Humility

It takes humility to be grateful for what we have in life, and thus it's a natural manifestation of a healthy mind and spirit. When I speak of humility, I am not speaking of timidity. If humility is genuine, it will be noticed by others, and not by us. It becomes part of who we are.

It takes a balanced, courageous person to be humble. Watch the degree of humility you feel on a daily basis, as it will indicate the shift from a balanced state of our spiritual level to an unbalanced state. If we find arrogance is rising, our humility is fading, and chances are that we are insufficiently balanced at the spiritual level.

4. Intensity of Love Toward Self and Others

Universal love is the unconditional acceptance of one's self, others, and life. Unconditional acceptance requires letting go of our expectations. The ability to manifest this aspect presupposes a person who is well-balanced in the intelligences above this level (physical, mental, and emotional). It requires emotional stability, mental balance, and excellent physical condition.

Love results from feeling joy and trust at the same time. If we find ourselves experiencing sadness, disgust, or remorse, we are low in manifesting love. Monitoring our ability to unconditionally love our self, fellow humans, and animals allows us to gauge any shift at this level.

If there is a change, it indicates that there is a change in our balanced state. Lack of unconditional love manifests as being judgmental or finding fault with others. It is a sign of our own incompleteness, and therefore indicates an imbalanced state. Only a person with a balanced spiritual level can express unconditional love.

5. Degree of Contentment and hope

Hope is what engages us with the spiritual level. If we want to be connected with our spiritual level, we need to experience hope regularly. When a person is well-balanced at the spiritual level, they feel content, and hopefulness manifests automatically.

There is a big difference between contentment and happiness. Happiness results from selfish gain, and therefore relies on external input and is not permanent. Contentment, on the other hand, results through acts of selfless giving, and arises from a balanced and unwavering spiritual level within us.

At the Unknown Level

This intelligence connects to us by producing a sense of "being" experienced while awake. The "being" relates to the sense of being alive or sense of existence in this world. This is the level of the universal intelligence—our true self in contrast to the description of our personality—fake self. Not a lot is known about this level, as it is uniquely individual to each person. We mentally connect with this level through faith. Religion can have influence in the faith at this level. However, religion is not necessary for one to experience faith in universal intelligence. This sense is spontaneous in everyone. This level is present in atheists and agnostics too.

The unknown level is where the universal intelligence operates. This universal intelligence is very elusive due to its intangibility to our conscious awareness. This level generates the other four intelligences that are part of our inner self, and those intelligences become more and more tangible as we ascend toward the physical level (Figure 18.3). The two characteristics that I describe below go hand in hand when it comes to recognizing our being at this level.

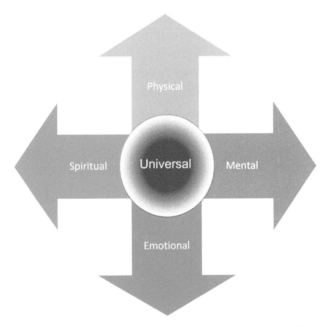

Figure 18.3: The five intelligences of our inner self.

1. Intensity of Faith

Faith is optimistic by nature; it is associated with expectation of positive outcomes but its foundation is unwavering trust. Faith, belonging to unknown level, gives rise to hope belonging to spiritual level. Faith and hope are intricately intertwined because spiritual intelligence is the immediate and closest manifestation of the universal intelligence.

There is a big difference between true hope associated with a realistic sense of optimism, and false hope associated with an unrealistic sense of optimism. We all hope to win the lottery, but only a few do. In this case, there is no realistic plan for winning beyond buying the ticket. In most cases, however, we can come up with a realistic plan for achieving what we are hoping for.

The first key element is to determine whether we feel realistically optimistic toward whatever we are engaged in. The second key element is whether all five intelligences are completely aligned with the hope, and without even the slightest bit of doubt—faith.

The "realistic" component is a vulnerable area because our rationalization and silent partner has influence here. Our rationalization and silent partner can work against alignment of all intelligences toward a said outcome. Faith has the power to align and bind all intelligences together and channel these intelligences to rely on our true being. I've seen patients whose recovery was doubted by entire groups of physicians walk out after a major illness because of their intensity of faith. On the other hand, I've also seen us destroy the elements of faith-related alignment and resulting hope in patients by medical transparency. For example, telling a patient that they have six months to live without providing an avenue for faith to operate can result in the patient's intelligences working against each other. These patients never made it out of the hospital. There is nothing wrong with medical transparency, but when and how we deliver that news should be considered, so as not to destroy a patient's faith in them. Further yet, I have also seen patients with rationalization and false hopes reject medical recommendations. These patients like Mr. Priest are no longer with us.

Monitoring the intensity of realistic hope indicates the strength of our connection with, and faith in, the universal intelligence. The less balanced we are, the less connected we are with the universe, and the less hopeful we become. As discussed before, when the doorway to the unknown/universal level shuts, life ends.

2. Ability to Sustain Uncertainty

Are you someone who needs to have all your ducks in a row before embarking on a plan of action? Can you take a leap of faith? The ability to take a leap of faith in uncertain circumstances comes from our strength of connection with the universe. It reflects an ability to function without having everything understood in clear terms. As a result, the ability to function under uncertain circumstances requires faith. It's therefore easy to monitor this manifestation of the unknown level by detecting changes in our level of hope and our connection with the unknown intelligence. As mentioned before, our strength of connection depends on our balance in the other intelligences, which are all generated from the universal intelligence (Figure 18.3).

It is evident that the descriptions of each level's balance-indicators change from being more tangible to less as we descend through the levels of the BMIT. This is important to recognize. There is little power in tangibility, and great power in intangibility. Previously, we've discussed that we function from all levels of the BMIT, but we tend to linger on one level, depending on which intelligence predominates our life.

The key to success depends on whether we can function from the unknown level—the most powerful of all intelligences. I call it functioning in the grey zone, as it is the zone of uncertainty (it's neither black nor white). When we force our self to function in this zone, we engage with "realistic hope" (as opposed to "unrealistic hope," which is like wishful thinking) and are taking a leap of faith. Realistic hope at spiritual level is how we connect to the unknown level and faith anchors us to the universe.

CHAPTER 19

Rule #6: Renew health daily

Cultivating Ability

There is an old story about the tree and the grass. The big, strong tree stood like a mountain in the jungle. During the day, several animals took refuge in its shadow to escape the heat. At night, birds and animals called it home. A few feet from the tree was a patch of grass. One day, the tree was insulting the grass as to how weak, small, and useless it was, compared to the tree's strength, size, and ability to provide for the animals of the jungle.

The grass replied, "I can withstand insults because I am small and pliable."

The tree laughed at the grass, and said, "That's no skill compared to being a mighty being like me."

That night, a furious thunderstorm, with gushing winds as never seen before, descended on the jungle. The next day, there were dead animals and fallen trees everywhere. The grass, peeling itself away from the ground, stood up and looked around. The big and strong tree was nowhere to be seen. The grass finally found it lying on its side, uprooted from the ground, dying. The grass said to the tree, "How did your size and strength help you with what happened last night?"

The tree said, "You are still alive, and I am dying."

Health is ability and it's one that requires accumulation and careful maintenance of precise skills. These skills in turn prepare us to being responsive to changes and being ready to respond at any given time. Being healthy is not avoidance as we did during the pandemic of 2020. Avoidance is precaution. Being healthy relates to preparedness. That readiness requires continuous rebalancing, which involves renewal. Chapter 12 discussed two types of renewal: *spontaneous renewal* and *cultivated renewal.* Our body carries out spontaneous renewal of vital-force without any active input from us. The human body is inherently designed to perform this action for survival. *The vital-force is the most potent medicine there is.* We can positively facilitate and influence both renewals of vital-force in three ways:

1. By choosing actions that facilitate the body's spontaneous renewal process.
2. By avoiding actions that impair the body's ability to spontaneously renew.
3. By taking additional actions that purposefully promote cultivated generation of vital-force and increase our health reserve.

Actions that promote spontaneous renewal or result in the generation of additional vital-force are called *health assets.* In contrast, actions that impair spontaneous renewal or deplete our vital-force are called *health liabilities.*

In the words of financial educator and bestselling author, Robert Kiyosaki, "Anything that puts money in your pocket is an asset and anything that takes money out of your pocket is a liability." However, even with liability, there is "good" and "bad" liability. A "good liability" is one that requires a little money out of our pocket initially, but appreciates over time and results in a bigger long-term return on investment, like purchasing a rental property. On the other hand, a "bad liability" is something that depreciates in value, like a car.

In health, vital-force is the equivalent of money to wealth. Therefore, *anything that puts vital-force into our body is a health asset and anything that takes vital-force out of us is a health liability.*

A health liability does not always have to be an action. It can be as simple as a lingering negative emotion like anger or being upset. It could be any conflict within us.

Just like in wealth, there are good and bad liabilities in health, too.

A "good liability" is something that turns out to be an asset in the long run. This is a habit that requires an initial investment of vital-force, but provides an appreciative increase in the return on that investment, like regular exercise. Our body also spontaneously uses "good liability," like when digesting food. It takes energy to digest and absorb food, which in turn provides more energy than what was spent to digest it.

A "bad liability" is something like the habit of smoking. Smoking causes expenditure of vital-force to counter the adverse influence of smoke on lung tissue, but it gives no appreciative return in the form of vital-force. One could argue that smoking helps alleviate anxiety or nervousness. This argument concerns using smoking as a distraction for an already existing problem, but when we use an action to alleviate a problem, it becomes a crutch. Thus smoking is a wrong coping skill for that problem. A suitable remedy for nervousness or anxiety would be to identify the cause of the ill-feelings and actively work on solving that cause. This is in contrast to a masking action, like smoking, which is depreciative for health, and therefore a health liability.

Upon learning he had a life-ending disease, Mr. Addict chose to undergo drug rehabilitation. He didn't choose drugs to counter the anxiety from his diagnosis, though he could have. He chose to be like the grass—responsive to change. I've encountered patients plunging into the same bad habit that produced their bad situation in the first place. These patients had a weak silent partner and were not willing to strengthen it. Winners use corrective actions, and thus assets, to counter bad situations. They learn how to be responsive. Losers use masking actions, and thus liabilities, to counter bad situations, and ultimately perpetuate the bad situation. Losers resist and refuse to be responsive.

What You Can Do and Use

Winning in health means understanding health assets and liabilities, and training to be responsive when a change in the balance between them is recognized. In accordance with the 3R formula (Recognize, Rebalance, Remain Balanced), renewal relates to rebalance. Rebalancing works best when it is a daily habit, just like we discussed in Chapter 14.

There are several functions that are liabilities, but that are nevertheless essential for living (items A, B, and C; Figure 19.1). There are others, however, that are non-essential for living (item D; Figure 19.1). Choosing to avoid those non-essential liabilities, or converting them to health assets, is one way to increase the strength of non-renewable vital-force—the reserve. This non-renewable portion automatically becomes available when we need to engage an invisible enemy, like COVID-19. That is the secret of those that survived the pandemic and those that have overcome other life-threatening diseases. Smart people minimize or eliminate non-essential liabilities from their daily life, add health assets, and choose to engage in "good" liabilities.

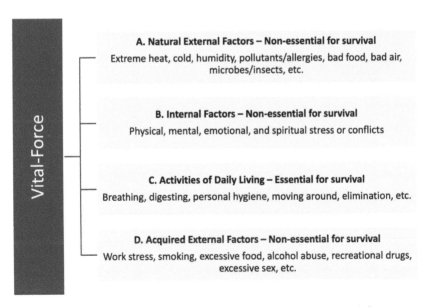

Figure 19.1: Examples of health liabilities in our daily life.

As explained above, there are those actions that are necessary for the basic activities of daily living, called essential health liabilities, and those that are not necessary but we choose to engage in anyway. Just as there are health liabilities, which we choose to engage in, there are health assets that we can also engage in. Essentially any activity, modality, feeling, or mood that puts more vital-force into our inner self is a health asset, and anything that takes energy out of us is a health liability.

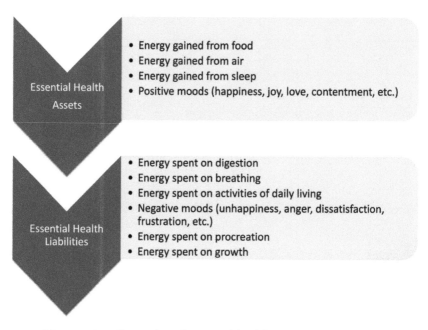

Figure 19.2: Examples of essential health assets and liabilities.

Figure 19.2 describes examples of essential health assets and liabilities. They are called essential based on whether they are needed for our survival or not. Once the concept of health assets and liabilities becomes clear, the next step is to invest our daily actions on assets and minimize actions that are liabilities. Essential health liabilities cannot be avoided but can be influenced to be "good liabilities" with effort (Figure 19.3). The table below provides examples of ingredients required for renewal of vital-force and sources for obtaining those ingredients.

Physical level Vital-force renewal What is required	Physical level Vital-force renewal What you can do
✓ Proper diet	✓ Clean balanced diet
✓ Proper exercise	✓ Regular exercise
✓ Proper breathing	✓ Yoga/Tai Chi/clean air
✓ Proper hygiene	✓ Detoxification/physical cleanse
✓ Proper rest	✓ Fasting ✓ Ensure 7-9 hours sleep

Table 19.1: Requirements and resources for vital-force renewal at the physical level.

Mental & emotional level Vital-force renewal What is required	Mental & emotional level Vital-force renewal What you can do
✓ Create positive attitude	✓ Meditation
✓ Create positive emotions	✓ Time for self-reflection
✓ Create positive stress	✓ Emotional cleanse
✓ Create positive actions	✓ Yoga/Tai Chi

Table 19.2: Requirements and resources for vital-force renewal at the mental and emotional level.

Spiritual & universal level Vital-force renewal What is required	Spiritual & universal level Vital-force renewal What you can do
✓ Creating contentment	✓ Selfless giving
✓ Being true to yourself	✓ Time for self-reflection
✓ Engaging the spirit	✓ Meditation

Table 19.3: Requirements and resources for vital-force renewal at the spiritual and universal level.

Convenience versus Inconvenience

We live in a world of conveniences. Conveniences steal our vital-force. Earlier, we discussed the action of eating food as a good liability. It is a liability because it requires an initial investment of vital-force to digest, absorb, and distribute the nutrients. It is "good" because those absorbed nutrients give us more vital-force in return than we initially lost. In the end, the return on investment is positive. However, this isn't always the case, and ultimately it depends on what food we eat.

Take fast food for example, which often contains fats, oils, preservative chemicals, hormones, and antibiotics. Additionally, the food is cooked in a way that depletes it of micronutrients. Our body has to invest a lot of energy to digest and absorb all these fats and chemicals, and the food doesn't have a lot of nutrients to begin with. As a result, the return on investment of that food is low, if any, making it a "bad" liability. On the other hand, consider a meal that contains fresh vegetables, fruits, and lean meat without preservatives or chemicals. It is easy to digest and has more nutrients, and the return on investment is greater, making it an asset. Examples of other essential liabilities and how to convert them to "good" liabilities are given in Figure 19.3 below.

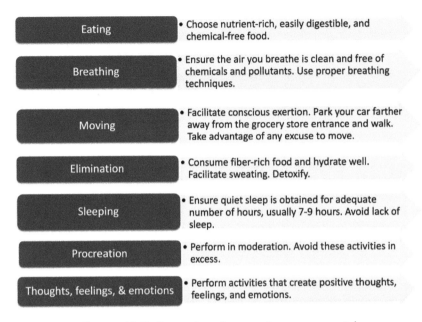

Figure 19.3: Examples of converting our essential liabilities to good essential liabilities.

The goal of renewability, however, is not to make us all become vegan. If we choose to be vegan, good for us, but it's not necessary. All that is required is the knowledge and mindfulness to recognize that consumption of a particular food can be a liability. Once recognized, rebalance is accomplished through carrying out a cleansing process or correcting the liability with health assets for the next few meals. Eating bad food once in a while is not an issue, but having no awareness of it, making a habit of it, and not using corrective action is an issue.

The requirements and sources given in the figure above for vital-force renewal are designed to address all five levels of our inner self. It is important to pick daily actions that address all of the levels in order to maintain balance. Using what we discussed in Chapter 18 with regard to recognizing health transitions will enable us to adjust the degree of renewal actions that need to be carried out.

CHAPTER 20

Rule #7: Maintain lifelong health

A nything dynamic requires continuous effort. The ability to maintain balance of our inner self—called health—is no different. In the previous chapter, we discussed continuous renewal. Renewal relates to what we can do ourselves to generate and maintain the balance between health assets and liabilities. This balance in turn determines life-flow, and life-flow in turn determines health status. Continuous positive life-flow helps preserve the non-renewable portion of vital-force, which is our health reserve.

Mind the Gap

While rebalancing is an individual effort, maintaining health involves using our health team. This chapter relates to the "remain balanced" portion of the 3R formula, which is about designing and executing a pattern of regular interaction with the members of our health team to have them monitor, recognize, and advise on rebalancing our inner self.

Even with utmost diligence, our chronological aging, environmental influences, and daily stressors creep up and steal our vital-force. As a result, biological aging continues. While it is possible to recognize the transition from "H" quadrant to "I" quadrant, it is incredibly difficult to become an expert on it unless we dedicate a considerable amount of time. The health team steps in to fill the gap created by our lack of personal time. Our ability to reserve time to maintain health determines how wide or narrow the gap is. The bigger the gap, the more frequently one will require the services of the health team.

There are some people who are so busy pursuing their goals that they have no time to invest in their own health. In this situation, a team becomes extremely important. I have known very successful individuals who failed in health, simply because they failed to build the right health team. These individuals were very savvy in creating winning teams to achieve other goals, but they failed to create a health team until it was too late.

There are others who are busy in a different way. They're not in pursuit of big goals, but of making ends meet in their life. As a result, they don't have spare time for adopting a healthy lifestyle. There're two major barriers for these people: lack of time and lack of money. This leaves health on "autopilot," where the body's spontaneous renewability (Chapter 19) is the sole contributor to their health. This is a one-person team, and it's insufficient for staying healthy.

A third group of people neither pursue higher goals nor try to make ends meet. A multitude of factors in life conspire against this group making them unable to put time and work in and instead, lean on the world to keep them upright. This group of people is already unhealthy. In this instance, the health is not only left to spontaneous renewal but also is actively damaged. Having a health team is not even on their radar.

Irrespective of group, class, or creed, everyone deserves to be healthy. All of us can become healthy and maintain a lifestyle that promotes health and minimizes the occurrence of disease. Small steps go a long way and cumulative effect of our actions is real. The key is getting started.

1. Start with augmenting the spontaneous renewal process of the body to enhance the generation and minimize the expenditure of vital-force.

2. Once Step 1 becomes a habit, add on other actions that are health assets to begin forming a reserve of vital-force—cultivated renewal.

3. Once Steps 1 & 2 become habit, it is key to ensure that healthy actions, habits, and lifestyle are maintained.

This last process serves to fill the gap created by our lack of personal time, and this is when we engage our health team for monitoring, check-ups, or therapy.

The process is similar to caring for a house. We protect it with regular maintenance, and have a team of people to help us maintain it. For example, we have a handyman, an electrician, a plumber, a landscaper, a pool service, a bricklayer, etc. We don't always need them, but they are there to help when we do.

Managing the generation (health assets) and expenditure (health liabilities) of vital-force is a daily task, and it's dependent on the individual. The balance we create between health assets and health liabilities determines positive or negative life-flow leading to respective healthy state or ill-health over time. Despite daily effort, life-flow can be affected by factors out of our control, such as natural biological aging. This requires periodic inspection and careful monitoring.

Life-flow maintenance What is required	Life-flow maintenance Team member involved	Life-flow maintenance Tools used
• Regular disease/ screening (annual)	• Modern medical practitioner • Anti-aging/Metabolic medical practitioner • Naturopath	• Physical exam • Blood tests • Imaging tests
• Regular health screening (every 3 months)	• Complementary/Eastern Medical practitioner • Chiropractor • Acupuncturist • Iridologist • Naturopath	• Homeopathic assessment • Chiropractic assessment • Iris analysis • Traditional Chinese medicine
• Optimize biological aging (every 3 months)	• Anti-aging /Metabolic medical practitioner	• Anti-aging therapy • Hormone balance • Stem cell • Botanicals • Vitamins
• Physical cleanse (every 6 months)	• Complementary/Eastern medical practitioner • Anti-aging/Metabolic medical practitioner	• Dietary detox
• Emotional cleanse (every 6 months)	• Psychological counselors • Psychiatrists	• Psychological counseling • Biofeedback • Hypnosis
• Energy balance (every month)	• Complementary/Eastern medical practitioner • Acupuncturist • Massage therapist • Herbalist • Reflexologist • Spiritual therapist	• Acupuncture • Aromatherapy • Botanicals/Herbs • Color therapy • Massage therapy • Music therapy • Pet therapy • Reflexology • Spiritual therapy

Table 20.1: Basic requirements, team members, and tools used for health maintenance.

The above table lists the basic requirements for maintenance of life-flow. The minimum frequency is what's required for a reasonable balance of our inner self. This frequency may change based on life-flow direction (positive vs. negative), or based on how busy we are. Change in frequency does not always require a visit to a team member, but indicates an interaction with the team member. The team members are our teachers and coaches.

Stress is the single most frequent disrupter of our inner self. It affects us by disrupting the balance of our emotional intelligence. Remember—emotion is energy in motion. Subsequently, disrupted emotion leads to disruption of vital-force, which unbalances our life-flow. Emotion resides at the center of the five intelligences of our inner self. This is because emotion plays a major role in success and failure in any of life's undertakings, which is why the energy balance requirement in the table above is to be cared for more frequently than others. Fortunately, we have a lot of tools available for us to handle our emotional intelligence.

As a practicing heart transplant cardiologist, the importance of having a team became evident after witnessing its impact on patients in life-or-death situations. Later reflection confirmed that the absence of a health team played a prominent role in the progression of my own coronary artery disease. Even as a physician-expert in both Eastern and Western medicine, I failed in health at age forty-four, simply because of a failure to mind the gap created by the lifestyle of a physician. Even though I had all the necessary knowledge about health and disease, I had no time to take action based on that knowledge. In fact, I neither practiced the steps described in this book nor did I have a team at the time of my heart attack. Knowledge leads to nowhere if no action is taken. A simple, but a frequently overlooked idea.

In modern life, it's easy to fail to recognize the importance of a health team and succumb to the health gap. Most of us grow up with such a team when we are children, albeit less members than what is proposed in this book (pediatrician, dentist, swim coach, baseball coach, soccer coach, dance teacher, music teacher, etc.), but that team dissolves when we become adults. As adults, most of us fail to form teams in any endeavors we undertake, including health, and wonder why we fail.

CHAPTER 21

Rule #8: Recruit an expert advocate

Need for Guidance

A fifty-year-old woman was in a medically-induced coma and supported with machines to treat her failing heart. This was the first time she had been hospitalized with any medical problem in her life. Her loving husband sat by her every day and witnessed all the doctors come by and care for her. They also communicated to him what they thought was best for her, based on their assessment of her progress.

I was one of the physicians taking care of his wife and giving a daily update on her progress. Watching him, one could appreciate the love he felt for her, as well as the pain of being forced into an incomprehensible situation. Although the husband was her medical power of attorney, they had never discussed a situation like this—they hadn't foreseen it as a possibility at such a young age. Medically, she was actually making progress, but none of the machines were being removed, because her condition was still not strong enough.

All the husband could see was that his loving wife remained unconscious. She was unable to communicate, and the medical jargon was overwhelming him. Since he couldn't communicate with her, he chose the next best people for help; his family, friends, and priest. There was no medical professional among them.

I walked in one morning to find that the family was preparing to withdraw all support from the patient and let her pass on. This was devastating; as my professional opinion was that the patient could recover if given enough time for her internal environment to rebalance itself on life support. We were in a conundrum: the medical professionals thought the patient's internal environment had not yet reached the point of no return, but her husband, family, and friends made the emotional decision to let her go. The difference; family judged by the outward appearance of the patient and medicine judged by the appearance of the internal environment.

In modern medicine, we accept a decision, irrespective of whether the driver of that decision is our mental, emotional, or spiritual intelligence. These concepts are not included in modern medicine's disease care. Modern medicine also does not question the subjective or objective nature of the decision. This story emphasizes the importance of an expert advocate when we encounter disease. It is the same with building health and a health team. Obviously, the primary champion of your team is you. However, there needs to be a secondary advocate in your team, as well.

As we continue to educate ourselves on health, and work toward that goal, our ability to be an efficient champion gradually increases. But the very increase in our ability also increases our bias toward ourselves. That's why we still need an objective secondary health advocate; our health education only sharpens our ability to pick the right one.

This expert advocate is like our handyman. Whenever there's an issue with our house, the handyman recommends whether we need an electrician, plumber, etc. They are aware of all aspects of what is happening in the house. Likewise, our health advocate provides similar services while educating us in health.

Remember, our team members are those who sell their services to us and are experts in certain fields only. There are some who may have enough working knowledge of other specialties to guide us, even though they do not provide those services. Our health advocates should at least have broad knowledge of all areas of health along with awareness of their own limitations, so that they can point us toward the specific specialty or specialist we need to consult with. In addition, our health advocate should also be our mentor at a time of decision-making, just like the patient-story described at the beginning of this chapter.

The Right Health Advocate

For most people, health advocates are their primary care physician, naturopath, homeopath, or complementary/alternative medical practitioners. There is nothing wrong with any one of them, as long as they are open-minded and have the best interest of our health driving their advice. One thing to keep in mind is to be skeptical if an advocate, whether a modern physician or complementary practitioner, criticizes other disciplines that they are uneducated about. A modern physician that has no concept of complementary health cannot possibly judge those practitioners. Likewise, an alternative physician, who has never stepped into a hospital, cannot judge a modern physician's ability to care for disease.

There is a saying: "A razor blade is sharp, but can't cut a tree; the axe is strong, but can't cut a hair. Everyone is important according to their own unique purpose." The problem starts when the razor blade tries to be an axe, and vice versa. If we witness this among our team members, it is time to find another team member.

I've witnessed disastrous outcomes in patients due to such an attitude from their practitioners. There was a fifty-year-old man with heart failure who only sought help from an alternative medical practitioner. He subsequently withered away and died at age fifty-one due to a misdiagnosis. Likewise, I've seen several patients who were not directed to seek alternative or complementary therapies for diseases which modern medicine has no treatment for, and they suffered a poor quality of life as a result.

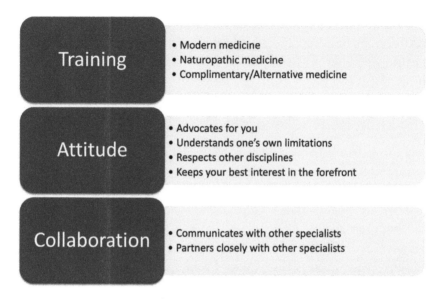

Figure 21.1: Basic characteristics of an expert health advocate.

From birth, we grow up with people guiding us. Initially, our parents are our guides and mentors, providing constant support through early childhood. Later on, we may add schoolteachers, leaders of the scouts, and priests as our guides. If we play sports, we add our coaches also. Once we become adults, these guides fall by the wayside, and we find more guides in our peers, but less in number. Transitioning into adulthood, we increasingly engage our silent partner as our guide to solve problems and less of other mentors. When we rely on our silent partner for success, the outcome depends mainly on the coping skills of the individual. Most of us are not actively taught appropriate coping skills as we grow up.

We start solving our problems by ourselves because that is how our education system trained us. We forget to function as a team, and more importantly, we forget about our guides. We become our own advocates and rely on our silent partner to deliver. The problem is, our silent partner is only as good as what it has been exposed to.

The range of exposure of our silent partner to information on health is negligible. An average person's exposure to health education at home and school during the stages of childhood and young adulthood is mostly about disease. The silent partner does not have adequate and appropriate rules of function when it comes to health. As a result, our silent partner is not an expert in health. This is the reason health isn't on our radar until disease strikes, and it's the reason we need a health team and a health advocate. With our team's guidance, we continue to educate ourselves in health. A team-based approach with the correct views and concepts places us at an advantage to be winners.

CLOSING THOUGHTS

Congratulations!

Reaching this far is the hardest. If you have survived this far, you have learned to say "no" to your silent partner. You are stronger than your silent partner. You have also made health personal to you. You are now equipped with six different views, seven thought-provoking concepts, and eight rules to conduct a successful journey towards being a winner in the space of health. Here are the key takeaways:

- ✓ Health is an *ability* – It can be cultivated
- ✓ Health system is *disease* care – Function outside of it
- ✓ *Balance* is the single focus of health – It's nature's law
- ✓ Currency of health is *energy* – It's already in your possession
- ✓ Health is *renewable* – It can be individually accomplished
- ✓ Health is *dynamic* – it's a lifestyle
- ✓ *Aging* is inflation in health – It can be slowed
- ✓ *Silent partner* is our barrier – It can be modified
- ✓ Health is a *team effort* – It's the key to success
- ✓ *Spirit* drives health – It can be recruited

Thinking different is the single most important attribute to personal success. The above key takeaways are different than what is currently thought about health in society at large—and is perhaps even diametrically opposed.

Next Steps

A goal without a plan is just a wish.

Start your journey by reading this book as many times as necessary to make the views and concepts your own. Start with simple steps that are achievable. Create a reward system and give yourself a pat on the back for reaching small goals. Once a decision for commitment is made, your first step is to self-cleanse, which facilitates change through neuroplasticity and awareness of the silent partner. This newly cultivated mindfulness of your silent partner allows you to get closer to your inner self where the spirit resides. The next step is learning how to develop a habit. The cumulative benefit you receive from these two steps is the initial goal, which will take time to manifest based on your individual timeframe. As it manifests, the progress will be expedited. As progress becomes perceptible, the process becomes rewarding. A habit is then developed which becomes your lifestyle—a healthy lifestyle.

Remember the health code?

"I commit to a lifestyle of health by creating a team, and adopting self-cleansing to engage my spirit to recognize, renew, and maintain my health with guidance."

Effort is your responsibility...

A Personal Guide

Survival depends on success
Success depends on effort
Effort is fueled by knowledge
Knowledge comes from discovery
Discovery is through imagination
Imagination originates from humility
Humility requires courage
Courage comes from love
Love originates in spirit
Spirit is universal and the key to successful survival
All of these naturally exist within you
Commit to; JUST BE YOU
SUCCESS WILL FOLLOW

-Radha Gopalan, MD

END NOTES AND CITATIONS

Caplan, A.I. (2007), Adult mesenchymal stem cells for tissue engineering versus regenerative medicine. J. Cell. Physiol., 213: 341-347. https://doi.org/10.1002/jcp.21200

Cowan, & S. F Morall (2020). *The contagion myth: Why viruses (including "coronavirus") are not the cause of disease.* New York, NY: Skyhorse Publishing.

Homeostasis: Definition of Homeostasis by Oxford Dictionary on Lexico.com also meaning of Homeostasis. (n.d.). Retrieved from https://www.lexico.com/en/definition/homeostasis

Huber, M., Knottnerus, J. A., Green, L., van der Horst, H., Jadad, A. R., Kromhout, D., Leonard, B., Lorig, K., Loureiro, M. I., van der Meer, J. W., Schnabel, P., Smith, R., van Weel, C., & Smid, H. (2011). How should we define health?. *BMJ (Clinical research ed.)*, *343*, d4163. https://doi.org/10.1136/bmj.d4163

Lally, P., van Jaarsveld, C.H.M., Potts, H.W.W. and Wardle, J. (2010), How are habits formed: Modelling habit formation in the real world. Eur. J. Soc. Psychol., 40: 998-1009. https://doi.org/10.1002/ejsp.674

Late Sequelae of COVID-19. (2020, November 13). Retrieved from https://www.cdc.gov/coronavirus/2019-ncov/hcp/clinical-care/late-sequelae.html

Liester M. B. (2020). Personality changes following heart transplantation: The role of cellular memory. *Medical hypotheses, 135,* 109468. https://doi.org/10.1016/j.mehy.2019.109468

Neuroplasticity. (n.d.). Retrieved from https://www.psychologytoday.com/us/basics/neuroplasticity

Ornish, D., Lin, J., Daubenmier, J., Weidner, G., Epel, E., Kemp, C., Magbanua, M. J., Marlin, R., Yglecias, L., Carroll, P. R., & Blackburn, E. H. (2008). Increased telomerase activity and comprehensive lifestyle changes: a pilot study. *The Lancet. Oncology, 9*(11), 1048–1057. https://doi.org/10.1016/S1470-2045(08)70234-1

Rediger, MD, J. (2020, May 06). Your Immune System is Your Greatest Asset-Here's How to Care For It. Retrieved from https://elemental.medium.com/your-immune-system-is-your-greatest-asset-heres-how-to-care-for-it-4356cee6598c

Sartorius N. (2006). The meanings of health and its promotion. *Croatian medical journal, 47*(4), 662–664.

Segerstrom, S. C., & Miller, G. E. (2004). Psychological stress and the human immune system: a meta-analytic study of 30 years of inquiry. *Psychological bulletin, 130*(4), 601–630. https://doi.org/10.1037/0033-2909.130.4.601

Skin. (2017, January 17). Retrieved from https://www.nationalgeographic.com/science/article/skin-1

Taylor, B. (2018, April 10). What Breaking the 4-Minute Mile Taught Us About the Limits of Conventional Thinking. Retrieved from https://hbr.org/2018/03/what-breaking-the-4-minute-mile-taught-us-about-the-limits-of-conventional-thinking.

Thacker, S. B., Stroup, D. F., Carande-Kulis, V., Marks, J. S., Roy, K., & Gerberding, J. L. (2006). Measuring the public's health. *Public health reports (Washington, D.C. 1974), 121*(1), 14–22. https://doi.org/10.1177/003335490612100107

Witze, A. (2016). Unseen planet may lurk near Solar System's edge. *Nature, 529.* https://www.nature.com/news/polopoly_fs/1.19182!/menu/main/topColumns/topLeftColumn/pdf/529266a.pdf?origin=ppub

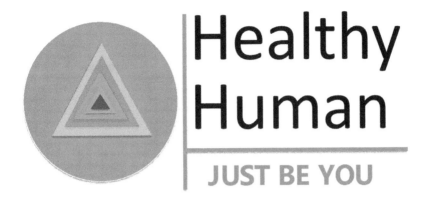

Healthy Human

JUST BE YOU

One Simple Mission:
Elevating Individual Health

One Simple Philosophy:
A human being is complete. Medicine is incomplete.
Optimal health is achieved by combining all
medicines with the power of the spirit.

One Simple Claim:
You Are the Medicine

One Simple Effort:
Just Be You

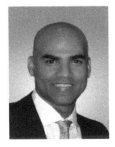 *"The health of a person is not defined by the presence
or absence of disease. It is rather defined by the ability
of the individual to get back to the balanced and
optimal state from derangement, and maintain that
balance at all levels that constitute a human being."*
—Radha Gopalan, MD

www.healthyhumaneducation.com
 @healthyhumaneducation

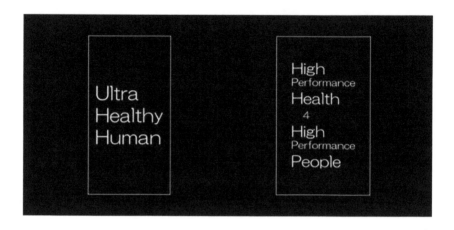

Ultra Healthy Human

High Performance Health 4 High Performance People

The Latest in Medical Technology, for a Younger, Sexier, Energized, You

Dr. Nicole Srednicki, DNP, ABAAHP
Personalized, Anti-Aging & Integrative Medicine

Dr. Radha Gopalan, MD

Scottsdale, Arizona
480-699-4242

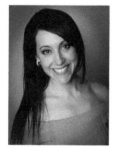

"Human aging begins at birth. A toxic physical and mental environment accelerates this very process. Being ultra-healthy is a lifelong process of converting these liabilities into assets. How a person accomplishes this is an individual choice."
-Dr. Nicole Srednicki

www.ultrahealthyhuman.com
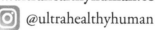 @ultrahealthyhuman

OTHER BOOKS BY DR. RADHA GOPALAN

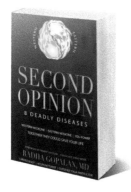

CHANGE THE WAY YOU
THINK ABOUT YOURSELF—
AND MEDICINE—FOREVER

LEARN WHY BEING HEALTHY
HAS MORE TO DO WITH
WHO YOU MUST BE THAN
WHAT YOU MUST DO

Dr. Radha Gopalan, gifted heart transplant cardiologist, addresses the confusion and mixed medical messages related to health, wellness, and illness from a unique and powerful perspective that blends his experiences with both Eastern and Western medicine. He delivers not only concepts and personal stories that can change the way you think about health and wellness, but also assesses the most common medical conditions that impact our world—from obesity and cancer to lung, liver, kidney, and heart disease.

The book was born from 30 years of seeking answers to some intriguing—and sometimes troubling—observations of people, disease, diagnosis, health, current trends in healthcare systems, and spirituality. In *Second Opinion*, Dr. Gopalan explains:

- How Eastern and Western medicine can work together for optimum health and wellness
- How your power can shape your personality, reactions, health, and happiness
- Why some people who eat healthy, exercise, and lead a healthy life have heart attacks.
- Why your health is affected more by who you are than by what you do

. . . .

"Without health there is no wealth, and Dr. Gopalan teaches us who we must be to stay healthy.
He's an important part of my own personal health and wellness team and my good friend."
Robert Kiyosaki

. . . .

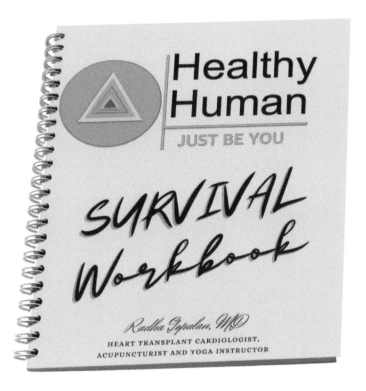

Don't just read–learn!

Download the FREE Survival workbook from
www.healthyhumaneducation.com/survival-workbook
and test your understanding of health.